Decision Making in Midwifery Practice

Edited by

Maureen D Raynor RMN RN RM ADM PGCEA MA

Midwife Teacher, University of Nottingham, School of Human Development, Academic Division of Midwifery, Post Graduate Education Centre, Nottingham City Hospital, Nottingham, UK

Jayne E Marshall MA RGN RM ADM PGCEA

Midwife Teacher, University of Nottingham, School of Human Development, Academic Division of Midwifery, Post Graduate Education Centre, Nottingham City Hospital, Nottingham, UK

Amanda Sullivan BA(Hons) PGDip PhD RM RGN

Consultant Midwife, Antenatal Clinic, Nottingham City Hospital NHS Trust, Nottingham, UK

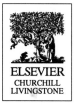

ELSEVIER
CHURCHILL
LIVINGSTONE

EDINBURGH LONDON NEW YORK OXFORD PHILADELPHIA ST LOUIS SYDNEY TORONTO 2005

ELSEVIER
CHURCHILL
LIVINGSTONE

An imprint of Elsevier Limited

First published 2005

ISBN 0 443 07384 8

British Library Cataloguing in Publication Data
A catalogue record for this book is available from the British Library

Library of Congress Cataloging in Publication Data
A catalog record for this book is available from the Library of Congress

Note

ELSEVIER your source for books, journals and multimedia in the health sciences

www.elsevierhealth.com

Transferred to Digital Printing 2009

The publisher's policy is to use paper manufactured from sustainable forests

Decision Making in Midwifery Practice

For Elsevier:

Commissioning Editor: Mary Seager
Development Editor: Rita Demetriou-Swanwick
Project Manager: Anne Dickie
Designer: Judith Wright

Contents

Contributors

Rosalind Bluff PhD SRN SCM ADM MTD CertEd
*Lecturer in Midwifery, University of
Southampton, School of Nursing and Midwifery,
Southampton, UK*

Elizabeth R Cluett PhD MSc RM RGN PGCEA
*Lecturer in Midwifery, University of
Southampton, School of Nursing and Midwifery,
Southampton, UK*

Pauline Cooke MSc RGN RSCN RM ADM PGCEA
*Consultant Midwife, St Mary's Hospital NHS
Trust, London, UK*

Jean M Duerden MBA RM RN RSCN
*LSA Midwifery Officer, Yorkshire and Northern
Lincolnshire LSA, West Yorkshire Strategic
Health Authority, Leeds, UK*

Professor Shirley R Jones MA RGN RM ADM
CertEd (FE), Teaching (Midwifery), SoM ILT
*Head of School of Women's Health Studies,
University of Central England, Birmingham, UK*

Dr Sally Marchant PhD RM RN DipEd
Editor, MIDIRS Midwifery Digest, Bristol, UK

Jayne E Marshall MA RGN RM ADM PGCEA
*Midwife Teacher, University of Nottingham,
School of Human Development, Academic
Division of Midwifery, Post Graduate Education
Centre, Nottingham, UK*

Marianne Mead RGN RM Ecole des Cadres (Brussels)
ADM MTD BA(OU) PhD
*Principal Lecturer and Associate Research
Leader, Department of Nursing and Midwifery,
University of Hertfordshire, Hatfield, UK*

Heidi Mok MSc PGCEA ADM SCM SRN
*Senior Midwifery Lecturer, Institute of Nursing
and Midwifery Education Centre, University of
Brighton, Pembury Hospital, Tunbridge Wells,
Kent, UK*

Kathleen P Nakielski MSc PgDipEd BA(Hons)
ADM RM RGN
*Midwife Teacher, University of Nottingham,
School of Human Development, Academic
Division of Midwifery, Mansfield Education
Centre, Nottingham, UK*

Maureen D Raynor RMN RN RM ADM PGCEA MA
*Supervisor of Midwives, Midwife Teacher,
University of Nottingham, School of Human
Development, Academic Division of Midwifery,
Post Graduate Education Centre, Nottingham, UK*

Jeanne Siddiqui MPhil CertEd RGN RM ADM
*Retired Midwife and Lecturer. Previously Head
of Midwifery Education, University College
Chester, Chester, UK*

Peggy A Stevens RN RM ADM PGCEA MSc
*Senior Midwifery Lecturer, Institute of Nursing
and Midwifery Education Centre, University of
Brighton, Pembury Hospital, Tunbridge Wells,
Kent, UK*

Amanda Sullivan BA(Hons) PGDip PhD RM RGN
*Consultant Midwife, Antenatal Clinic, Nottingham
City Hospital NHS Trust, Nottingham, UK*

Vicky Tinsley RN RM BSc (Midwifery)
MA (Industrial Relations)
*Maternity Services Manager, Trowbridge
Maternity Hospital, Trowbridge, Wiltshire, UK*

Acknowledgements

We are grateful to the contributors for their unstinting efforts, hard work and commitment in making this publication a reality. A special thank you is extended to Rosalind Bluff for her visionary ideas and sharp intelligence in generating the proposal and laying the foundations for this ground-breaking textbook, to her we are truly indebted.

Introduction

Maureen D. Raynor and Rosalind Bluff

INTRODUCTION

Decision making is a fundamental and integral part of professional practice; decisions that are made will determine the actions as well as practice of the midwife and the quality of midwifery care. Historically, midwives have not been renowned for using evidence to make informed and rational decisions. Even when they have concerns they do not always question the decisions made by others such as general practitioners or junior medical staff (Lewis and Drife 2001). This, coupled with the constraints of the medical model of care, have culminated in midwives relying on doctors to make decisions for them (Garcia and Garforth 1989), and resulted in a reluctance to diffuse the power in their relationship with women (Kirkham 2000). More recently, decision making has become increasingly important as changes have taken place not only within the maternity services but also within the National Health Service (NHS) as a whole, making the provision of care more complex and demanding. Clinical reasoning is therefore important to diagnose problems and facilitate decision making. This chapter will introduce the subject of decision making, along with key terms that are frequently used interchangeably when discussing this concept. The importance of decision making will be highlighted, and a guide on how to use the book provided.

AIMS/PURPOSE OF THE BOOK

Midwives can no longer expect to rely on policies and protocols devised by doctors to determine their practice (Symon 1998). The culture is changing, and there is now an expectation that midwives will make decisions within evidence-based guidelines, using their professional judgement. How these decisions are made – and the factors that influence the midwife's decision making – are therefore of paramount importance and need to be made explicit. The purpose of this book is to provide a philosophical debate and decision-making frameworks aimed at increasing midwives' awareness of the process of decision making in professional practice. The ultimate goal is that the utilisation of these frameworks will facilitate or enhance practice and improve the quality of care offered to child-bearing women. It is also hoped that midwives will be encouraged to reflect on, and learn from their own practice. In this way they will be able to improve the professional judgements they make. Although the book is written primarily for midwives and students of midwifery, the principles and philosophy are transferable across professional boundaries. Thus, it may also be of help to other professional groups who have a concern to provide quality maternity care or health services in other healthcare settings. Care has been taken to ensure that the frameworks underpinning the book can be readily applied and utilised in practice. Consequently, practical examples are provided throughout the text that firmly root the theoretical paradigms to practice. Midwives act as role models and also have a responsibility in helping students learn how to make decisions. The visionary approach of this book will assist practitioners to make explicit to students how they make decisions, and in so doing empower and support students to develop the confidence to become accountable, reflective, autonomous practitioners.

THE IMPORTANCE OF DECISION MAKING IN MIDWIFERY PRACTICE

Successive reports from the Department of Health (DoH) such as 'Making a Difference' (DoH 1999), 'The NHS Plan' (DoH 2000a) and 'An Organisation with a Memory' (DoH 2000b), have all placed emphasis on accountability and autonomy in the context of healthcare. The ubiquitous report 'Changing Childbirth' (DoH 1993) heralded the majority of the change in current day maternity care. Much emphasis has been placed on creative ways of thinking and innovative ways of working such as working towards achieving one-to-one care (McCourt et al. 1998) and working sensitively with women via patterns of care, for example, caseload holding and group practices (Page 2000). The primary aim is to achieve woman-centred care with midwives acting autonomously and involving women in the decision-making process. Consequently, decision making is shared through working in partnership with women, colleagues and service providers. New roles have also been established around firm leadership such as the creation of midwife consultants, and other specialist posts to provide care for specific groups of individuals such as women with known vulnerability factors. These include domestic violence (DoH 2000c), diabetes mellitus (Scottish Intercollegiate Group Network [SIGN] 2001), female genital mutilation (Mwangi-Powell 2001), drug abuse (Lewis and Drife 2004) and refugees/asylum status (Burnett and Fassil 2002, James 2003). These new ways of organising and developing midwifery care have meant that increasing numbers of midwives are working in challenging and multi-complex ways, taking on more responsibility, fulfilling their autonomous role and providing total care for women. Furthermore, that responsibility extends to performing specialised skills such as ventouse extraction and examination of the newborn, a pre-condition of which requires midwives to make decisions and accept responsibility for their actions.

Midwives are accountable for what they do or do not do (Nursing and Midwifery Council 2004). Reports by the Department of Health (DoH 1998, 1999) have helped to widen the traditional boundaries of midwives' professional accountability in order to improve and maintain the quality of care and services provided to mothers and babies. Here, quality assurance has an important role involving risk management, auditing, and clinical effectiveness through the provision of evidence-based practice, that is, clinical governance. All of these factors have resulted in a dynamic and evolving role which means that more decisions must be made. Midwives are no longer just charged with providing care, they also have to be responsible for effective use of resources. The rapidly evolving role of the midwife and the culture in which she practises demands strong leadership. In its vision for the future of the maternity services, the Royal College of Midwives (RCM 2000:14) has set a standard of leadership that is 'visionary enough to risk radical change and accountable enough to allow women's views to shape and monitor the maternity services of the future'. Implicit within this standard is a requirement for confident and effective decision making.

Situations to which professionals apply their practice are often complex because they involve people (Higgs and Jones 2000, Higgs and Titchen 2000). Women have their own knowledge beliefs, cultural background, experiences, and perceptions. Yet decisions determine the quality of care that women receive. If inappropriate decisions are made, these can adversely affect the well-being of the mother and baby. Decision making is therefore associated with risk (Orme and Maggs 1993), and in an increasingly litigious society it is hardly surprising that some midwives are afraid of taking these risks (Symon 1998, Dimond 2002). Moreover, the hallmark of good decision making is not only crucial in refuting claims of negligence, but also the risk of negligence claims may be minimised in the first instance (Price 1995). Hence, there is a need for midwives to understand not just the decisions they make, but the process of making those decisions based on rational thought, analysis and reflection. This understanding means that decisions can be justified and others facilitated and supported so that they too can have confidence in their own ability to make informed and ethical decisions.

In their professional capacity, midwives act as role models and educators for students. Although traditionally students have not played an active part in the decision making process, if they are to learn how to become autonomous practitioners such skill needs to be transparent (Fraser et al. 1997, Cioffi 1998). Benner (1984) identified that expert practitioners make decisions based on intuition. If intuition is tacit knowledge that cannot be articulated this raises an issue about how students will learn to make their own decisions.

WHAT IS A DECISION?

A decision can be viewed from a number of perspectives. Jenkins (1985) defines decision making in terms of the process that begins with a problem or situation associated with inconsistencies that need resolving. Decisions can, however, be made in the absence of any problem and may involve choosing from a number of alternative options, courses or action (Baumann and Dauber 1989, Edwards and Elwyn 2002). Making a decision can therefore also be viewed from the perspective of an outcome, or alternatively as outcome and process. Women whose pregnancy is classified as 'low risk' may not have problems – just options regarding aspects of care. For instance, they can choose where they give birth (Midirs 2003, National Institute of Clinical Excellence [NICE] 2003) – for example, a midwifery-led unit, hospital, home or a private maternity centre. The existence of such options means that a decision must be made. In the absence of any option no choice can be made and there can be no decision (Cooke and Slack 1991). Moreover, Jennings and Wattam (1994) claim that the options from which a choice can be made would be expected to have different outcomes. When considering the options, the value of the outcomes therefore has to be considered (Baumann and Dauber 1989). This for example could relate to a woman who is deemed 'low risk' deciding whether to have a planned vaginal birth or an elective Caesarean section.

Lund and Robinson (1993) make a distinction between decision making and decision taking. Decision making is a process that involves gathering information, analysing and evaluating it while decision taking is the final step in this process. Conversely, Cross (1996) views the decision as the point at which a course of action is determined. Thus, the process of decision making is ongoing, commencing before the decision is made and continuing after the decision has been taken.

PROBLEM SOLVING

When the term *problem* is included in the definition of a decision it is not surprising that decision making and problem solving are sometimes viewed as being synonymous. Problem solving, according to Cooke and Slack (1991) and Danerek and Dykes (2001), is a broad process which includes identification and understanding of a problem, setting objectives, identification and evaluation of options, choosing an option, and implementing it in action. Decision making is primarily concerned with choosing between the available options. This supports the view of Barwell and Spurgeon (1993), that while making decisions is a crucial activity in management it is the problem-solving activities that support the decision making. Curiously, when the focus is shifted to solving problems the emphasis is on the outcome and not on the process of clinical reasoning. For the purposes of this book, the term *decision making* will be employed, but it should be remembered that many of the women for whom midwives provide care, do experience problems, and that those problems need to be recognised if appropriate decisions are to be made.

MAKING JUDGEMENTS

Closely linked to making decisions are the terms *clinical judgement* and *professional judgement*. Professional judgement requires the midwife to review the knowledge she has of all relevant aspects of the situation, and to choose the action that will achieve the desired goal (Price 1995). The decisions which midwives make as they fulfil their professional role, and the process involved in making those decisions, are both incorporated within professional judgement. Knowing what data to collect, its significance and establishing whether that data fits patterns of existing knowledge, are all part of that process (Gordon et al. 1994). Using professional judgement is just one skill involved in the decision-making process, but critical thinking or clinical reasoning is also a crucial component (Dowie and Elstein 1988).

Axten (2000) believes that making judgements and decisions is not about practitioners having power and control but recognising that women have needs, and they too should be involved in the process.

CRITICAL THINKING

Thinking is a cognitive process which enables all aspects of an issue to be examined from a number of perspectives (Paul 1993, Edwards 1998). To critically think means that in the process of exploring all perspectives, both the strengths and weaknesses of each view point will be considered. This involves having an internal dialogue with oneself to question what is done and how it is done. Critical thinking then becomes a purposeful activity designed to facilitate the decision-making process, and is important for midwives who are required to base their practice on evidence.

CLINICAL REASONING

Higgs and Titchen (2000:23) claim that: 'in the health professions, clinical reasoning provides the vehicle for knowledge use in clinical practice as well as for knowledge generation'. Alfaro-Lefevre (1995) sees 'reasoning' as a synonym for critical thinking, an essential skill central to the practice of professional autonomy. Clinical reasoning and knowledge are therefore interdependent. Higgs and Jones (2000) present clinical reasoning as a process that includes cognition, knowledge and the ability to monitor and adjust the thinking process. Thus, reflection facilitates thinking about cognition and enhances self-awareness. As Mong-Chue

(2000) asserts, knowledge on its own is not sufficient for making decisions, there is a need for a balance between knowledge, the pregnant woman's wishes and the midwife's clinical experience – in other words, evidence-based practice (Sackett 1997). Clinical reasoning consequently accounts for the context in which care is given and the wider context with women involved in decision making, and working collaboratively with service providers.

Gordon et al. (1994) convey nurses' reasoning as a form of clinical judgement that occurs in the following sequence: meeting the patient, gathering clinical information, generating potential diagnoses, determining the diagnosis, and making a decision about what action to take. Ritter (1998) views clinical reasoning as a process that includes evidence to facilitate optimum patient outcomes. Therefore nurses' clinical reasoning can be defined as the cognitive processes and strategies that they use to understand the significance of client data, to identify and diagnose actual or potential problems, to make clinical decisions to assist in problem resolution, and to achieve positive patient outcomes. Similarly, midwives deal with complex situations often filled with uncertainty. Decision making is not an exact science and requires many skills, including reflective practice and clinical reasoning (Schön 1987).

Pyles and Stern (1983) 'constructed a nursing Gestalt' to explain the cognitive process in decision making. The nurse links the current situation to a past experience, identifies cues from the client and sensory cues (described as gut feelings) to make decisions. Therefore, decisions could be based on a feeling rather than a thought. Orme and Maggs (1993) state that it is impossible to analyse intuitive practice, and any attempts to do so makes it a cognitive issue which ceases to be intuitive.

YOUR PRESENT APPROACH TO DECISION MAKING

The skills required to make decisions are having the ability to comprehend, interpret, analyse and synthesise data and the skills of inquiry. Readers are therefore invited to complete the reflective activity below to identify how they make decisions and then compare this with the different approaches presented in this book.

Reflective Activity

Are you conscious of making decisions?
Do you know how you make decisions?
Do you postpone making a decision?
Do you avoid making decisions? If so why?
   Are you afraid of the consequences?
Does your philosophy of practice correspond
   to the decisions you make?
How do your peers influence the decision
   you make?
Do you rely on others to make decisions for you?

HOW TO USE THE BOOK

The book can either be read from cover to cover, or each chapter can be examined individually. To achieve the aims of the book, a broad perspective of decision making has been adopted. Each chapter focuses on a specific aspect related to decision making. In Chapter 1, the concept of autonomy is explored. An historical perspective of the midwife's role is provided and the factors which enhance or inhibit the midwife's ability to make decisions and practise autonomously are considered.

A sound and developed knowledge base is a prerequisite for effective decision making (Orme and Maggs 1993). Decisions cannot be made unless the midwife has knowledge she can use to inform her practice. Chapter 2 examines the role of knowledge in decision making, the types and sources of knowledge, and their influence on practice. Knowledge that is regarded as evidence is detailed in Chapter 3, along with how it can be interpreted and used to inform decisions. The distinction is made between research-based practice and evidence-based practice.

The complex nature of midwifery practice means that there is no single approach to decision making. According to Barwell and Spurgeon (1993), some individuals stress the rational scientific 'step-by-step' approach to decision making. The traditional or rational approach is explored in Chapter 4. Others stress the importance of the 'art' of decision making by focusing on instinct, experience and judgemental flair. Both have their place, and Chapter 5 presents the challenges to decision making, while Chapter 6 discusses how professional judgement is developed.

Decisions are often associated with moral issues. Resolving dilemmas is not easy. The principle of autonomy says that individuals should be able to perform whatever actions they wish, presumably even if it involves considerable risk to themselves and others consider the action to be foolish (Beauchamp and Childress 2001). This may mean there is conflict between the interests of the mother and interests of the fetus, or the midwife has concerns that the actions of the mother may be detrimental to her or her baby. Chapter 7 examines the ethical theories that may be used to help resolve these dilemmas, coupled with the support available to midwives when coping with conflict.

Many midwives will be concerned about making decisions regarding how they care for mothers and babies, but decisions made by managers are more related to resources, contracting, cost-effectiveness, and so on. Responding to demands for change within the NHS and the need to provide woman-centred maternity services requires proactive clinical managers with strong leadership skills. Chapter 8 focuses on the different types of

decisions that managers have to make, and how quality can be achieved through consensus decision making. In Chapter 9, emphasis is placed on working in partnership with women and their families, and how women can be helped to make decisions in order to retain their own autonomy. Learning from practice can be facilitated through a process of reflection, and Chapter 10 addresses the concept and philosophies of reflection and how these can enhance decision making. Midwifery supervision places great emphasis on the provision of support for midwives in the fulfilment of their role. Chapter 11 teases out the ways in which supervisors of midwives can facilitate effective decision making and enhance the quality of midwifery care. The book concludes with Chapter 12, which reviews and summarises the main themes of previous chapters, making links between each one and their interface with midwifery practice.

In order to facilitate learning, a very practical approach has been adopted. All contributors are midwives with considerable experience. This will enable theory to be robust and credible, effectively applied to midwifery practice whilst ensuring that the content is up to date and of high quality. Each chapter is fully referenced and, where appropriate, suggestions for further reading are provided. Practice examples, activities, figures, flow charts and/or diagrams are used whenever indicated both to simplify the text and to assist with explanations and reflection on practice. Key points for best practice are provided at the end of most chapters to act as a quick reference guide for the reader. A glossary of terms is also included at the end of the book.

References

Alfaro-Lefevre R 1995 Critical Thinking in Nursing: A Practical Approach. WB Saunders, Philadelphia.

Axten S 2000 The thinking midwife arriving at judgement. British Journal of Midwifery 8(5): 287–290.

Barwell F, Spurgeon P 1993 Information for Effective Management Decision-Making in the NHS. Longman, Essex.

Baumann A, Dauber R 1989 Decision making and problem solving in nursing: an overview and analysis of relevant literature. Literature Review Monograph, Toronto University, Toronto.

Beauchamp TL, Childress JF 2001 Principles of Biomedical Ethics, 5th edition. Oxford University Press, New York.

Benner P 1984 From Novice to Expert. Addison Wesley, London.

Burnett A, Fassil Y 2002 Meeting the health needs of refugee and asylum seekers in the UK: an information and resource pack for health workers. Department of Health, London.

Cioffi J 1998 Education for clinical decision making in midwifery practice. Midwifery 14(1): 18–22.

Cooke S, Slack N 1991 Making Management Decisions, 2nd edition. Prentice-Hall, Hertfordshire.

Cross RE 1996 Midwives and Management: a Handbook. Books for Midwives, Cheshire.

Danerek M, Dykes A-K 2001 The meaning of problem solving in critical situations. British Journal of Midwifery 9(3): 179–186.

Department of Health 1993 Changing Childbirth: report of the expert maternity group. HMSO, London.

Department of Health 1998 A First Class Service Quality in the New NHS. The Stationery Office, London.

Department of Health 1999 Making a Difference. The Stationery Office, London.

Department of Health 2000a The NHS Plan. The Stationery Office, London.

Department of Health 2000b An Organisation with a Memory. The Stationery Office, London.

Department of Health 2000c Domestic Violence: a Resource Manual for Health Care Professionals. Department of Health, London.

Dimond B 2002 Legal Aspect of Midwifery, 2nd edition. Books for Midwives/Elsevier Science, London.

Dowie J, Elstein A (eds) 1988 Professional Judgement: a Reader in Clinical Decision Making. Cambridge University, Cambridge.

Edwards S 1998 Critical thinking and analysis: a model for written assignments. British Journal of Nursing 7(3): 159–166.

Edwards A, Elwyn G 2002 Evidence-based Patient Choice. Open University Press, Oxford.

Fraser DM, Murphy R, Worth-Butler M 1997 An outcome evaluation of the effectiveness of pre-registration midwifery programmes of education (the EME project). ENB, London.

Garcia J, Garforth S 1989 Labour and delivery routines in English consultant units. Midwifery 5(4): 155–162.

Gordon M, Murphy C, Candes D, Hiltunen E 1994 Clinical judgement: an integrated model. Advances in Nursing Science 16(4): 55–70.

Higgs J, Jones M 2000 Clinical reasoning in the health professions. In: Higgs J, Jones M (eds), Clinical Reasoning in the Health Professions. Butterworth Heinemann, Oxford.

Higgs J, Titchen A 2000 Knowledge and reasoning. In: Higgs J, Jones M (eds), Clinical Reasoning in the Health Professions. Butterworth Heinemann, Oxford.

James J 2003 Refugee women. In: Squire C (ed), The Social Context of Birth. Radcliffe, Oxon: Chapter 6, pp. 93–106.

Jenkins M 1985 Improving clinical decision making in nursing. Journal of Nurse Education 26: 6.

Jennings D, Wattam S 1994 Decision Making an Integrated Approach. Pitman Publishing, London.

Kirkham M 2000 How can we relate? In: Kirkham M (ed), The Midwife–Mother Relationship. Houndmills, Palgrave, Chapter 11, pp. 227–254.

Lewis G, Drife J (eds) 2004 Confidential Enquiry into Maternal and Child Health; Why Mothers Die 2000–2002. Sixth Report of the Confidential Enquiries into Maternal Deaths in the UK. RCOG Press, London.

Lund B, Robinson C 1993 Managing Health Services Book 4. Decision Making. Open University Press, Milton Keynes.

McCourt C, Page L, Hewison J, Vail, A 1998 Evaluation of one-to-one midwifery: women's responses to care. Birth 24: 81–89.

Midirs 2003 Place of birth, informed choice leaflet No 10 Midirs in Collaboration with NHS Centre for Reviews and Dissemination, Bristol.

Mong-Chue C 2000 The challenges of midwifery practice for critical thinking. British Journal of Midwifery 8(3): 179–183.

Mwangi-Powell F (ed) 2001 Female genital mutilation–holistic care for women: a practical guide for midwives. Forward, London.

National Institute of Clinical Excellence 2003 Antenatal Care: routine care for the healthy pregnant woman. Clinical Guideline 6. NICE, London.

Nursing and Midwifery Council 2004 The Code of Professional Conduct: standards for conduct, performance and ethics. NMC, London.

Orme L, Maggs C 1993 Decision making in clinical practice: how do expert nurses, midwives and health visitors make decisions? Nurse Education Today 13: 270–276.

Page LA (ed) 2000 The New Midwifery: Science and Sensitivity in Practice. Churchill Livingstone, Edinburgh.

Paul R 1993 Critical Thinking: What Every Person Needs to Survive a Rapidly Changing World. Centre for Critical Thinking, California.

Price A 1995 Sound Choices: Part 3: decision making and negligence. Modern Midwife, August: 10–13.

Pyles SH, Stern PN 1983 Discovery of nursing Gestalt in critical care nursing: the importance of the gray gorilla syndrome image. The Journal of Nursing Scholarship XV(2): 51–57.

Ritter B 1998 Why Evidence-based Practice? CCNP Connection 11(5): 1–8.

Royal College of Midwives 2000 Vision 2000. RCM, London.

Sackett DL 1997 Evidence-based Medicine: How to Practice and Teach EBM. Churchill Livingstone, New York.

Schön D 1987 Educating the Reflective Practitioner. Jossey-Bass, San Francisco.

Scottish Intercollegiate Network Group Management of Diabetes in Pregnancy 2001 Guideline 55, section 8. SIGN, Scotland. www.sign.ac.uk.

Symon A 1998 The role of unit protocols and policies. British Journal of Midwifery 6(10): 631–634.

Chapter 1

Autonomy and the Midwife

Jayne E. Marshall

INTRODUCTION

This chapter will examine the complex concept of autonomy within the context of midwifery decision making. By first of all presenting an historical perspective of the role of the midwife, followed by definitions and variations of autonomy, and then discussing those factors that influence the midwife's ability to make her own decisions, it is anticipated that the content will serve as a challenge for midwives to further develop their existing personal autonomy. Scenarios from practice are included within the chapter for the midwife/student midwife to consider and reflect upon the extent of their personal autonomy when making decisions in midwifery practice.

As a concept, the term 'autonomy' is indeed very complex, with limited and somewhat flawed theoretical dimensions when applied to the nursing and midwifery professions. Whilst it has been recognised that autonomy is considered to be one of the hallmarks of a profession, it remains questionable as to whether midwifery (and even more so, nursing) can be truly considered a profession so long as the medical profession exerts a degree of control over midwifery practice. As professional groups have historically been predominantly male – for example, medicine, law and theology – such groups have been concerned in maintaining control which has consequently continued to affect the extent of the midwife's autonomy to make her own practice decisions

(Clark 2004, Donnison 1988, Rothman 1984, Oakley 1976). To determine to what extent midwives in present-day maternity care are able to demonstrate autonomy in decision-making, a brief resumé of the historical perspective of the scope of the midwife's role will now be discussed.

AN HISTORICAL PERSPECTIVE OF THE SCOPE OF THE MIDWIFE'S ROLE

Up until the beginning of the last century, midwifery was an integral part of working-class life and culture. The midwife was a known and trusted supporter of women, who attended the majority of those unable to afford medical fees. However, the role remained unorganised, with the uneducated working-class midwives continuing to practise freely the skills passed down through the generations. Midwifery skills were essentially non-interventionist. Tew (1990) discussed how the midwife was able to assist the woman to use her own reproductive powers to give birth naturally, without damage and without any controlling interferences from other parties. This is supported by the fact that in the mid-1870s about 70% of all births in England and Wales were attended by midwives, and took place in the home (Donnison 1988).

However, the high maternal and infant mortality and the lack of education and training of the female midwives were of increasing concern. In 1902, the first Midwives Act was passed after much opposition – particularly from the more militant midwives who feared that such an Act would involve midwives finally surrendering their autonomy to medical control. This Act finally recognised midwifery as having clinical features of professionalism and hallmarks of a profession, such as specified training, and the maintenance of a register along with the inspection of midwives. However, Heagerty (1997) relates that while the Act provided the power to reform midwifery practice, it also affected a change in the relationship between the midwife and the woman, as well as her relationship to the

working class as a whole, because her loyalty was then to her profession rather than to the community in which she practised.

Two decades later, in 1924, when the home birth rate was 84%, the midwife's autonomy and scope of practice was again challenged as the maternal and infant mortality statistics continued to be the driving force in initiating the policy of institutionalised childbirth (Campbell 1924). Furthermore, despite any substantial evidence, the Peel Report of 1970 (Maternity Advisory Committee 1970) recommended that there should be 100% hospital births, and that small isolated obstetric units be phased out and replaced by consultant and General Practitioner (GP) units in general hospitals. This not only finally denied women the choice regarding the place of birth, but also further threatened the midwife's autonomy and scope to practise within the community setting.

The formation of the National Health Service in 1948, thereby providing the public with free general healthcare – including maternity care, at the point it was delivered – further affected the scope of the midwife's role. As a result, a more rapid shift towards birth in hospitals and maternity homes was experienced, and by 1958 the home birth rate had fallen to 34%. Moreover, antenatal care was made available to all women. The GP became the first contact for the pregnant women, and this in turn limited the midwife's autonomy from the outset as she was now less able to discuss maternity care options with the woman and make appropriate care decisions. In 1974, a further influence on attempting to restrict the community midwife's freedom to practise was the National Health Service (Reorganisation) Act (HMSO 1973). This meant that hospital and community midwifery services were to be centralised and managed within the confines of the one organisation, namely within the hierarchical structures of the hospitals. Consequently, all midwives in the NHS, including the relatively autonomous community midwives, were subjected to such control.

The **scope** of the midwife's role in the 1970s was constantly under threat of continuing technological advances and increasing obstetric intervention, particularly during labour. Midwifery became a subordinate profession that was hospital-based and under the auspices of obstetricians, who were now considered the experts in childbirth. Towler and Bramall (1986) discussed how the midwife became more of the doctor's assistant and technician supporting interventions such as inductions of labour, cardiotocography, artificial rupture of the membranes and epidural analgesia. It was not only the majority of midwives that accepted the decisions made by medical staff without any challenge, but also the women.

There was, however, a small group of midwives who demonstrated their dissatisfaction with the state system and decided to opt out and return to a style of independent practice that would allow them greater autonomy and job satisfaction. As Hunter (1998) claimed, in the early 1980s it was only independent midwives who were fulfilling the complete role of the midwife and working as practitioners in their own right. Currently, due to the issues of financial insecurity and increasing insurance costs, the number of independent midwives remains small (Tyler 1996, Cassidy 1994). It must, however, be argued that such a midwife provides her peers with a working role model for ideal practice that is centred around the holistic model of care, and not the fragmented model experienced by so many midwives.

Since the mid-1980s, midwives and women have contributed towards driving maternity care back to its focus of normalising childbirth for those women who are classed as 'low risk'. This move was supported by the Winterton Report (House of Commons Health Committee 1992), followed by the Report of the Expert Maternity Group, namely 'Changing Childbirth' (Department of Health 1993). Furthermore, policy documents such as 'The New NHS: Modern-Dependable' (Department of Health 1997), 'First Class Service: Quality in the New NHS' (Department of Health 1998) and 'Making a Difference' (Department of Health 1999) have provided midwives with opportunities to demonstrate they are able to practise autonomously. Innovative developments such

as team midwifery, midwife-led clinics, midwife-led units to the more recent reintroduction of birth centres, have not only led to midwives regaining some of the territory of normal midwifery lost to the medical profession in the 20th century by reasserting their autonomy, but also increasing the choices available to women (Kirkham 2003, Saunders et al. 2000, Flint et al. 1989).

During the past decade, there have been a number of developments in the scope of the midwife's practice that have provided opportunities for some midwives to acquire certain para-obstetric and obstetric skills, such as undertaking ventouse deliveries, ultrasonography and intravenous cannulation. However, Stafford (2001) argues that although midwives may view this acquisition as important, as such specialised roles can provide a degree of short-term 'illusory autonomy', others are more sceptical and may feel the tension between what they were trained to do and what they are currently being asked to do. Consequently, they may also face conflict between their professional **accountability** and fulfilling the requirements of their employers. As Symon (1994) warned, such a limited vision of professionalism is heavily subjected to the managerial imperatives of performance and efficiency and is unlikely to lead to enhancing the midwife's autonomy. Midwives therefore need to consider their own boundaries of practice and decide which aspects of their role they value most, without losing sight of the fundamental role of the midwife in normal midwifery. Furthermore, they need to bear in mind McKay's (1997) view that some midwives fear such developments could transform midwives into low-class medics.

DEFINITIONS AND VARIATIONS OF AUTONOMY

When defining the term *autonomy*, words such as self-rule, self-support, self-sufficiency, liberty, freedom, power and **authority** all come to mind (Marshall and Kirkwood 2000). Beauchamp and Childress (2001) acknowledge that personal autonomy as being, at a minimum, self-rule where the individual is in control of their own life and free from both controlling interference from others and from limitations, such as inadequate understanding, that can ultimately affect making meaningful choices and decisions. The autonomous individual therefore acts freely in accordance with a self-chosen plan. However, as being in control of one's own liberty and freedom should also involve behaving in both a **rational** and **moral** way, it would be wrong to assume that autonomy and freedom are synonymous.

As Pollard (2003) purports, from her examination of the literature pertaining to autonomy, the concept is considered to be a personal quality that enables individuals to express its associated characteristics. These are summarised in Box 1.1.

When midwives make decisions in practice they should also be aware of the antecedents and consequences of autonomy that are summarised in Box 1.2 by Pollard (2003) from the literature she reviewed.

FREEDOM AND PERSONAL AUTONOMY

Whilst it is acknowledged that freedom does not imply liberal indulgence of personal desires in an attempt to minimise frustration regardless of the effects such decisions and actions may have on other persons involved, autonomy expects the individual to be able to rationalise their decisions and actions. In

> **Box 1.1 Associated Characteristics of Autonomy**
>
> 1. Determining the sphere of activity under one's control.
> 2. Having the right and capacity to make and act upon choices and decisions in this sphere.
> 3. Having this right acknowledged by others affected by or involved in these decisions.
> 4. Taking responsibility for decisions made.
>
> Reference: Pollard K 2003 Searching for autonomy. Midwifery 19(2):115.

> **Box 1.2 Antecedents and Consequences of Autonomy**
>
> *Antecedents Necessary for the Exercise of Autonomy.*
> 1. A situation exists in which a course of action is required and in which options are available.
> 2. There is a need for the situation to be assessed.
> 3. There is a need for a decision to be made and acted upon.
>
> *Consequences of the Exercise of Autonomy.*
> 1. Responsibility is taken for the decision made.
> 2. The right to have made the decision is accepted as valid by others involved in the situation (even if disagreeing with the decision itself).
> 3. Personal esteem and confidence increase.
>
> Reference: Pollard K 2003 Searching for autonomy. Midwifery 19(2):115.

addition to the individual's personal integrity, other variables such as the interests of others, societal laws and rules, as well as organisational rules and procedures can further threaten the extent of personal autonomy the individual can have when making a decision.

As Feinberg (1973) claimed, real freedom is synonymous with self-discipline and self-restraint where the individual becomes free to make decisions concerning a variety of possible courses of action, demonstrating that the person has accepted true responsibility. A decision made by an individual that is either **impulsive**ly or **compulsive**ly driven is both unfree and non-responsible, and would indicate that such an individual lacks personal autonomy and the freedom to choose to do otherwise.

CONSCIENCE AND PERSONAL AUTONOMY

When making a decision, demonstrating self-discipline would also incorporate the ability to act conscientiously by seeking to always do what is right. Garnett (1969) contrasts *traditional* and *critical* **conscience** in decision making. Whilst traditional conscience constitutes internalised indoctrinated moral values, critical conscience re-assesses previously held moral values in conjunction with continuous appraisal of the individual's moral conduct. Where reason and desire are in conflict, the conscience (or will) is called upon. If the will is weak, then desire will prevail, whereas whenever the will is strong then reason will ultimately over-rule the desire. The integrity of the personality therefore depends on the strength of the will and the capacity of the individual to exercise their critical conscience, holding beliefs with the courage of conviction and being free to make appropriate decisions: being free from impulsively or compulsively driven behaviour.

Activity 1.1

You are currently working on labour ward providing care for Jill, a 22-year-old primigravida who is 38 weeks' pregnant. Unfortunately Jill's partner, Richard, is unable to be at the birth as he is currently working abroad. Having provided continuity of carer from the time Jill was first admitted to the labour ward, you have developed a trusting relationship with her. Jill appears to be making good progress and just as your shift is about to end she expresses to you that she feels the urge to push. However, you had earlier agreed to meet with friends after work to go for a drink.

- What do you decide to do?
- Consider how you made the decision, reflect on how your personal desires may/may not affect your moral reasoning.
- To what extent was your decision impulsive/autonomous?

AUTONOMY AS AN ETHICAL PRINCIPLE

It is one thing to be autonomous and another to be respected as autonomous. To respect an autonomous person is to recognise and appreciate the person's capacities and capabilities, including the right to certain views, to make

certain decisions and take certain actions based on personal values and beliefs. Such respect for autonomy is an **ethical** principle, being an intrinsic value of **deontology** (see Chapter 7). However, to what extent an individual is allowed choice in making decisions depends on their ability to rationalise, reflect and make clear judgement.

PROFESSIONAL AUTONOMY

Whilst it is difficult to define autonomy within the complex context in which midwives work, Henry and Fryer (1995) recognise that at the minimum it involves the exercise of choice and the power to make and act upon decisions. Furthermore, Lewis and Batey (1982) state that the professional autonomy of the health professional is associated with the freedom they have to make discretionary and binding decisions consistent within defined boundaries of their clinical practice, together with the freedom to act on those decisions. The midwife by the nature of **statutory** legislation, is solely responsible for making decisions in relation to the maternity care of individual clients to whom she is assigned within the context of normality (NMC 2004a). No other person has the rightful power to change that decision. In addition, advice from others can legitimately be accepted or rejected as midwives are ultimately accountable for their client's care. Autonomy is therefore restricted to that for which the midwife holds authority from expert knowledge and position, such that the autonomous midwife practitioner both decides and acts on the decision she makes. Autonomy cannot be decision making alone, as the decision is the foundation for determining a specific action or no action at all. Accountability, authority and autonomy are therefore linked as the right to self-govern and make decisions about their own clinical practice is an essential part of midwives being accountable. However, the degree that midwives are able to demonstrate their autonomy when making decisions in clinical practice is variable, and depends on the extent of authority given to them by the organisation in which they work, as well as their own personal willingness to accept such freedom.

Before moving on to discuss further the factors that influence the autonomy of today's midwife when making clinical decisions, it is worth being reminded that the majority of midwives who were educated and trained in the last century, had also undertaken nurse training where compliance and obedience to the doctor was the norm (Siddiqui 1996). With this in mind, it is useful to examine how the doctor–nurse power relations have manifested over time within the hospital setting to then appreciate its effect on decision-making in midwifery practice.

STEIN'S DOCTOR–NURSE GAME

Although it was recognised by Stein (1967) that the relationship between the doctor and nurse was considered special and based on mutual respect and interdependence, nurses were still expected to be subservient to doctors as far as decision making was concerned (Porter 1991). In 1967, Stein described how doctors have traditionally had total responsibility for making decisions regarding the management of their patients. In guiding the doctor's decision, data would be obtained from a range of sources, including a medical history, clinical examination, laboratory reports and recommendations from other specialists. In addition, recommendations from the nurse were also considered of importance to making a decision, but the interaction between the doctor and nurse through which these recommendations were communicated and received was unique to which Stein referred to as 'The Doctor–Nurse Game'.

The game actually arose from attitudes shaped by doctors' and nurses' training. Unlike medical students, who learned to play the game after leaving medical school, student nurses learned to play it early in their training. The sexual identity of the players was also seen as perpetuating the doctor–nurse game: doctors being predominantly men and nurses being mainly women. There were therefore some elements of the game that reinforced male dominance and female passivity. Through their training, student nurses were taught that the doctor had infinitely more knowledge than they had, and thus he was to be shown the utmost respect. They also learned that making suggestions to doctors was equivalent to insulting and belittling them – that is, it was synonymous to questioning the doctor's medical knowledge and insinuating that he did not know what he was doing. In direct contrast, however, the student nurse was also told that she was an invaluable resource to the doctor and was duty bound to contribute suggestions for the patient's benefit. Therefore, when the nurse felt that a recommendation would be helpful to the doctor, she – like the doctor – was caught in a dilemma: she was not allowed to communicate it directly, nor was she allowed not to communicate it. Consequently, the doctor–nurse game was played.

The fundamental rule of the game was that open disagreement between the players must be avoided at all costs. Nurses therefore had to communicate their recommendations without appearing to be making them. Similarly, doctors requesting a recommendation from a nurse needed to do so without appearing to be asking for it, as the recommendation had to be seen to be initiated by the doctor. When the game was successful, the obvious reward was a doctor–nurse team that operated efficiently where the nurse was used by the doctor as a valuable consultant and consequently gained self-esteem and professional satisfaction, alongside the doctor who gained the respect and admiration of the nursing service.

The penalties for failure of the game, on the other hand, could be severe. Doctors who were unskilled gamesmen and failed to recognise the nurse's subtle recommendations were tolerated as idiots. Furthermore, the lives of those doctors who interpreted these messages as insolence and strongly indicated they would not tolerate suggestions from nurses, could be made unbearable by the nursing staff. On the other hand, nurses who were unskilled at the game equally suffered. The nurse who neither viewed her role as a consultant nor attempted to communicate any recommendations to the doctor, was perceived as ineffective and consequently was ignored by medical staff and allowed to fade into obscurity. In comparison, the outspoken nurse who saw herself as consultant, but refused to follow the rules of the game not only was made to feel disliked, but also her life was made unbearable by medical and nursing staff.

INTERACTION STYLES

A study by Porter (1991) into the power relations between nurses and doctors in a general hospital revealed four major types of interactions in decision making that are also worth considering by the midwife when making clinical decisions. These were:

* unproblematic subordination
* informal covert decision making
* informal overt decision making
* formal overt decision making on the part of the (nurse) midwife

Each will now be discussed in turn within the midwifery context of amniotomy as an attempt to highlight the midwife's autonomy in decision-making.

(i) Unproblematic Subordination

This is the traditional interpretation of the doctor–nurse interaction and involves the midwife's unquestioning obedience of medical orders and the complete absence of any midwifery input into the decision-making process. Instances where an obstetrician gives the midwife an order without prior consultation or explanation, where midwives carry out that order without further negotiation, and where no alternative explanation could be suggested for their apparent subservience would be classified as belonging to this type. Furthermore, this interaction would demonstrate a total lack of autonomy on the part of the midwife in the decision-making process as the following interaction demonstrates:

Practice Example 1.1

SHO: (examining the partogram). I think it best for you to rupture the membranes otherwise she'll be in labour all night.
Midwife: OK.

(ii) Informal Covert Decision Making

Informal covert decision making is based along the lines of Stein's doctor–nurse game, which involves the pretence of unproblematic subordination whereby the midwife would show respect for the obstetrician and refrain from any open disagreement with them or making direct recommendations or diagnoses, while at the same time attempting to have an input into the decision-making process. The situation where a midwife makes recommendations about a woman's condition as substitute, where the obstetrician requests or accepts recommendations in the same fashion, and where there are no other feasible explanation for their actions are classified in this group. It could be argued that the following interaction between the midwife and doctor also demonstrates a certain lack of autonomy on the midwife's part. It is ultimately the SHO who makes the decision for the amniotomy despite the subtlety of the midwife's recommendation.

Practice Example 1.2

Midwife: (to SHO) Chris!
SHO: Yes?
Midwife: Sarah (Client) hasn't made much progress since the last examination. Her membranes are still intact.
SHO: OK. You'd best get on and do an ARM.

(iii) Informal Overt Decision Making

In this type of interaction it is expected that the midwife will openly contribute to decision making on an informal basis by demonstrating the extent of her knowledge and critical thinking, which consequently demonstrates increased autonomy. As Porter (1991) discovered in his study, the more **assertive** the nurse was in challenging the doctor's orders, the more the interaction appeared to resemble that of unproblematic subordination, but on this occasion the doctor was in the subordinate role. The following interaction attempts to highlight this:

✓ Practice Example 1.3

SHO: Sarah (Client) hasn't made much progress, I want you to do an ARM.

Midwife: Well, she has been resting on the bed for quite a while now. We have discussed her getting up and mobilising for a while to see if that will improve her contractions. I can't really see a need at the moment for an ARM. Why don't we wait and see how things go in the next couple of hours?

SHO: That's fine. Examine her again in a couple of hours.

(iv) Formal Overt Decision Making

Within midwifery practice, the role that midwives play in decision making is not only enshrined in statutory legislation as far as normal midwifery is concerned, it is also formalised by the responsibility they have for record-keeping (NMC 2004a, NMC 2004b). A typical example would be the use of midwifery care plans that is formulated by the midwife with the woman, written up and revised according to the woman's needs/condition, as well as that of her baby. Such a scheme demonstrates the midwife's ability to independently assess the woman's/baby's needs, plan and implement the care, and then evaluate the care – making any modifications if necessary from the original plan. In this particular type of decision making, the midwife can demonstrate her autonomy, where she is free to make appropriate judgement without any interference from others. However, there will be situations where the midwife – by the nature of her expert knowledge – recognises a deviation from normal progress in either the woman's or baby's condition and makes the decision to consult with other appropriately qualified

personnel, medical or otherwise (NMC 2004a). Such an autonomous decision would also be reflected in the midwifery care plan. Applying the above to the scenario of amniotomy, an extract from the intrapartum midwifery care plan could read as follows:

✓ Practice Example 1.4

01:00: **On admission:** Contracting 4:10 lasting 40 seconds. On Palpation: Fundus = Term, Longitudinal Lie, LOL position, Cephalic Presentation 3/5 palpable. Fetal Heart 136 bpm. Vaginal examination: Cervix fully effaced, 5 cm dilated. Membranes intact. Discussed birth plan and Sarah (Client) wishes to keep them intact to avoid the need for any pain relief. Fetal Heart 140 bpm...

05:00: Sarah sleeping on bed. Contracting 3:10 lasting 30 seconds. Fetal Heart 138 bpm...

06:00: Sarah now awake. Contracting 2–3:10 lasting 30 seconds. Fetal Heart 140 bpm. Sarah asks how much longer her labour will last. Discuss that one way of finding out would be to do a further vaginal examination to assess her progress, but otherwise there is no indication. Sarah consents to the examination.

06:05: On Palpation: Cephalic Presentation 3/5 palpable. Fetal Heart 136 bpm. Vaginal examination undertaken: Cervix 7 cm dilated. Membranes intact. Fetal Heart 138 bpm. Discuss Sarah getting up and mobilising to aid descent of the presenting part and improve strength and frequency of contractions. Some progress made in the past 5 hours, but contractions not as strong as on admission. Alternative would be to rupture the membranes but this would increase Sarah's need for pain relief, and she wants to avoid both. Suggest review the situation in a couple of hours after Sarah has been mobile. Sarah agrees.

06:15: Sarah gets up and begins to walk around the birthing room. Informed Dr. O of this decision.

✎ Activity 1.2

You are a community midwife on call for the night. Joanne is 41 weeks' pregnant with her first baby and she contacts you as she has experienced spontaneous rupture of the membranes. However, apart from the occasional tightenings, she does not appear to be contracting.

* What do you decide to do?
* Considering the four types of interactions, reflect on how you made the decision.
* To what extent is your decision autonomous?

FACTORS INFLUENCING AUTONOMOUS DECISION MAKING

STATUTE

Recent changes to the statutory bodies governing the education and practice of nursing, midwifery and health visiting, have resulted in the formation of the Nursing and Midwifery Council (NMC) (Nursing and Midwifery Order 2001). With a more even representation of members across the three disciplines than in the former UKCC, as well as successfully retaining the Statutory Midwifery Committee, there is the potential that the new streamlined statutory body may show more interest in developments within the midwifery profession and the role of the midwife. Nevertheless, some sceptics may argue that until midwives have their own specific regulatory framework, the autonomous nature of midwifery will never be fully recognised. However, in comparison, it must be recognised that statutory legislation in the form of the midwives rules and standards, does support the midwife in making autonomous decisions in relation to the maternity care of women who are considered to be low risk (NMC 2004a).

THE EDUCATION AND PROFESSIONAL STATUS OF MIDWIVES

In the last decade of the 20th century, fundamental changes had taken place in the education and training of the future midwife along with the transfer of midwifery education from schools of midwifery into Higher Education Institutions (HEIs). There has been a move from the shortened pre-registration programmes for registered nurses to the widespread introduction of a 3-year 'direct-entry' programme leading to a diploma/degree in midwifery. The evaluation of these programmes has been widely documented through the Effectiveness of Midwifery Education (EME) project (Fraser et al. 1997) as far as competence to practice was concerned. However, Pollard's (2003) study, although small, comprising of only 27 midwives from the south west of England, found that those midwives who had been educated by the direct-entry route were perceived to be more capable of exercising autonomy in making practice decisions than were the nurse-trained midwives. This could be as a consequence of the new diploma and degree programmes with initiatives such **as Problem/Enquiry Based Learning (PBL/EBL)**. These developments have provided students with a greater depth and breadth of knowledge, research awareness and ability to be assertive and challenge practice with confidence than was the norm with the shortened certificate level programmes (see Chapter 2).

The move of midwifery education and training into HEIs has also provided midwives with increasing opportunities to study to degree and masters/doctorate level. However, there is a dilemma that although the academic level of midwifery education has improved tremendously over the past century, raising not only the professional status of midwives but also the status of women in general, there is still much work that needs doing to readdress the balance of birth being a normal physiological process. The development of modules on 'normality', advancing midwifery practice and Active Birth seminars, to name but a few, can serve as a means of inspiration to midwives to develop their autonomy in decision making. By reasserting confidence in their knowledge of the normal physiological processes related to childbirth alongside their clinical abilities, such continuing professional development activities could be the motivating force for midwives to consider when making autonomous decisions in practice.

INTERPROFESSIONAL LEARNING AND WORKING

Further social policy in the form of 'The NHS Plan' (Department of Health 2000), advocated the importance of health professionals working and learning together in partnership to break down the barriers that inhibit creative and best practice. This was extended in the Department of Health's (2001) policy document 'Working Together Learning Together', where partnership between NHS, HEIs and the regulatory/professional bodies was endorsed. Within the latter publication, the sharing of common and core skills particularly the development of communication skills, was highlighted as a means of gaining a better understanding of each health professionals' role in practice. Innovations such as **Interprofessional Team Objective Structured Clinical Examinations (ITOSCEs)** can assist student midwives and medical students in making decisions together as a team whilst at the same time recognising the full extent of each other's role (Symonds et al. 2003). As Marshall and Kirkwood (2000) claimed, the real change that is occurring among those providing maternity care, is in attitude – that is, whilst midwives appear determined to be thought of as autonomous practitioners, their medical colleagues now appear more willing to allow them to practise autonomously.

POLICIES, PROCEDURES AND GUIDELINES

National and local Trust policies and procedures affecting maternity care practice may either enable/inhibit the midwife to make autonomous decisions. This is dependent on such guidelines being formulated with midwifery representation. Jowitt (2001) states that **National Institute for Clinical Excellence (NICE)** guidelines affecting midwifery practice have been developed based on obstetric and paediatric principles rather than midwifery ones. It is here where the challenge therefore lies for midwives to assert themselves and gain a voice to not only support their own interests, but also those of the childbearing women. Whilst it is important that clients receive evidenced-based care as Dimond (2001) asserts, the development of such guidelines depends on who is evaluating the available research: this is where midwives could play a vital role (see Chapter 3).

ROLE MODELS

Midwives who are confident and assertive in decision making are considered ideal role models for both students and newly qualified midwives to emulate. Where students encounter midwifery practice in a range of midwifery settings other than that of the acute hospital, such as midwife-led units and birth centres where policies and procedures are totally woman-centred being formulated by midwives, they are more inclined to appreciate the full scope of the midwife's role and her ability to make autonomous decisions without the interference of others.

The type of clinical environment to which student midwives have been mostly exposed during their education and training therefore can play a substantial role in developing confident and autonomous decision-makers. Whilst some students are confident to take up work in birth centres and have their own caseload upon qualification, others who may not have had such experience, can easily become socialised in the medicalisation of childbirth embracing technology and intervention. In areas where midwives are indoctrinated in a medical model, the student will be less inclined to develop the skill of making autonomous decisions. Resources such as staffing levels and workplace pressures may not only inhibit the provision of effective mentorship and preceptorship (Meakin 2003), but also the midwife's freedom to make appropriate decisions with the woman.

In order to address this imbalance of clinical experience, in May 2003, the Royal College of Midwives (RCM) launched its strategy for midwifery education in the document 'Valuing Practice: a Springboard for Midwifery Education' (RCM 2003). Among many of its wide-ranging recommendations was for students to gain more experience of maternity care provision in the primary sector, such as the home, in birth centres and group practice midwifery, in order to encourage their development into autonomous practitioners. Although there currently may be resource implications to provide such midwifery based practices throughout all areas of the United Kingdom, the RCM recommendations are expected to serve as a challenge for midwives to take control of their education and make such a vision a reality within the next five years.

The creation of consultant midwife posts for midwives who have studied to masters/doctorate level, has also attempted to raise the social and professional profile of midwives. These consultants, especially those whose role focuses on normality, are in an ideal position to change the balance of power and assist midwives in establishing autonomy in practice and decision-making (O'Loughlin 2001). However, it could be argued that these consultant midwives have a particularly onerous task ahead with the possible likelihood of conflict arising with obstetricians regarding labour ward practices. In comparison, the consultant midwife with a health promotion/public health role, may find less conflict in fulfilling her role, particularly in those areas which the government have specifically targeted to be improved, for example, breastfeeding, teenage pregnancy and smoking. Whilst the consultant midwife, regardless of her role and area of expertise, should be an ideal role model for midwives and students to emulate regarding best practice and autonomous decision making, she is very much reliant on the midwives' support and their individual willingness to take responsibility for practice decisions in order to successfully lead the midwifery profession forward.

RESPECT FOR THE WOMAN'S AUTONOMY

Respect for the autonomy of the woman will have some effect on the decisions that the midwife makes (see Chapter 9). Where there is a good relationship between midwife and client, there is less likelihood of any conflict arising in respect of decisions made about midwifery care provided. Through the use of **reflection** (Johns 2000), challenges in decision making can be explored with students and midwives in the classroom setting/peer support groups as a means of increasing confidence in their decision-making abilities (see Chapter 10). It may also be a consideration for the midwife to always include the Supervisor of Midwives in those instances where a conflict of interest arises with the woman that consequently challenges the midwife's professional judgment and autonomy in making decisions (see Chapter 11).

Activity 1.3

As a community midwife you have provided care for Lisa throughout both her pregnancies. She has recently given birth to Christopher at home with your support and in the presence of her husband Alex and their 4-year-old daughter, Kate. Christopher was born at term weighing a healthy 3.8 kg.

When discussing with Lisa and Alex that their GP will visit them to undertake Christopher's neonatal examination once he is 24 hours old, the couple express that they want YOU to examine him rather than a doctor who they hardly know.

- What do you decide to do?
- Reflecting on the decision you made, to what extent was your decision autonomous?
- Which specific factors do you feel contributed to either enabling you or inhibiting you to make an autonomous decision in this situation?
- If faced with a similar situation, how could you demonstrate the full extent of your autonomy in making the decision?

CONCLUSION

This chapter has attempted to examine the complexities of the concept of autonomy by offering an historical perspective of the midwife's role and the many factors that enhance or inhibit the midwife's ability to make her own decisions. Through the use of realistic scenarios from practice, it has also attempted to facilitate discussion and debate by challenging the reader to reflect upon their own personal autonomy when making decisions in current day midwifery practice.

KEY POINTS FOR BEST PRACTICE

- The extent of the midwife's autonomy remains a contentious area of debate.

- Throughout the last century and up to the present day, the role of the midwife has been faced with many changes in practice that have consequently challenged this role and affected her ability to make autonomous clinical decisions.

- Autonomy expects the individual midwife to be able to rationalise the decisions they make regarding actions/omissions in clinical practice.

- Current statutory legislation supports the midwife in making autonomous decisions in relation to maternity care of women who are considered to be low risk.

- Interprofessional learning and working initiatives can help to break down barriers that inhibit creative and best practice, whilst also enabling the professional to appreciate fully the extent of each other's role in making clinical decisions.

- Midwives who are confident and assertive in decision making are ideal role models for student midwives and newly qualified midwives to emulate and lead the midwifery profession successfully through the 21st century.

References

Beauchamp TL, Childress JF 2001 Principles of Biomedical Ethics, 5th edition. Oxford University Press, Oxford.

Campbell JM 1924 Reports of Public Health and Medical subjects. HMSO, London.

Cassidy J 1994 Indemnity costs puts the squeeze on go-it-alone midwives. Nursing Times 90(2): 7.

Clarke R 2004 Midwifery autonomy and the code of professional conduct: an unethical combination? In: Frith L and Draper H (eds), Ethics and Midwifery, 2nd edition, Books for Midwives Press, Edinburgh, pp. 221–236.

Department of Health 1993 Changing Childbirth, Part 1: Report of the expert maternity group. HMSO, London.

Department of Health 1997 The New NHS: Modern-dependable. HMSO, London.

Department of Health 1998 First Class Service: Quality in the New NHS. HMSO, London.

Department of Health 1999 Making a Difference: strengthening the nursing, midwifery and health visiting contribution to healthcare. HMSO, London.

Department of Health 2000 The NHS Plan. HMSO, London.

Department of Health 2001 Working Together – Learning Together: a framework for lifelong learning for the NHS, HMSO, London.

Dimond B 2001 Legal issues: end of year review and some predictions for 2001. British Journal of Midwifery 9(1): 49–52.

Donnison J 1988 Midwives and Medical Men: a History of the Struggle for the Control of Childbirth. Historical Publications, London.

Feinburg J 1973 Social Philosophy. Prentice-Hall, New Jersey.

Flint C, Poulengeris P, Grant A 1989 Know your midwife scheme: a randomised trial of continuity of care by a team of midwives. Midwifery 5: 11–16.

Fraser DM, Murphy R, Worth-Butler M 1997 An outcome evaluation of the effectiveness of pre-registration midwifery programmes of education (the EME project). ENB, London.

Garnett CA 1969 Conscience and conscientiousness. In: Feinburg J (ed), Moral Concepts. Oxford University Press, Oxford, pp. 80–92.

Heagerty BV 1997 Willing hand-maidens of science? The struggle over the new midwife in early twentieth century England. In: Kirkham MJ, Perkins ER (eds), Reflections on Midwifery.

Baillière Tindall, London, pp. 70–95.

Henry C, Fryer N 1995 Organisational ethics: the ethics of care. In: Henry C (ed), Professional Ethics and Organisational Change in Education and Health. Edward Arnold, London, pp. 110–117.

House of Commons Health Committee 1992 Second Report: Maternity Services (The Winterton Report). HMSO, London.

HMSO 1973 The National Health (Reorganisation) Act. HMSO, London.

Hunter B 1998 Independent midwifery: Future inspiration or relic of the past? British Journal of Midwifery 6(2): 85–87.

Johns C 2000 Becoming a Reflective Practitioner: a reflective and holistic approach to clinical nursing, practice development and clinical supervision. Blackwell Science, Oxford.

Jowitt M 2001 Not very NICE: induction of labour: draft guidelines – a commentary. Midwifery Matters 89: 23–25.

Kirkham MJ (ed) 2003 Birth Centres: a social model for maternity care. Books for Midwives, London.

Lewis FM, Batey MV 1982 Clarifying autonomy and accountability in nursing service: Part 1. Journal of Nursing Administration 12(9): 13–18.

Marshall JE, Kirkwood S 2000 Autonomy and teamwork. In: Fraser D (ed), Professional Studies for Midwifery Practice. Churchill Livingstone, Edinburgh, pp. 127–141.

Maternity Advisory Committee 1970 Domiciliary and maternity bed needs (Sir John Peel: Chairman). HMSO, London.

McKay S 1997 The route to true autonomous practice for midwives. Nursing Times 93(46): 61–62.

Meakin S 2003 Education to save midwifery. MIDIRS Midwifery Digest 13(2): 157–160.

Nursing and Midwifery Council 2004a Midwives Rules and Standards. NMC, London.

Nursing and Midwifery Council 2004b Code of Professional Conduct: standards for conduct, performance and ethics. NMC, London.

Nursing and Midwifery Order 2001 SI 2002 253. HMSO, London.

Oakley A 1976 Wise woman and medical men: changes in the management of childbirth. In: Mitchell J, Oakley A (eds), The Rights and Wrongs of Women. Penguin, Harmondsworth.

O'Loughlin C 2001 Will the consultant midwife change the balance of power? British Journal of Midwifery 9(3): 151–154.

Pollard K 2003 Searching for autonomy. Midwifery 19(2): 113–124.

Porter S 1991 A participant observation study of power relations between nurses and doctors in a general hospital. Journal of Advanced Nursing 16: 728–735.

Rothman B 1984 Childbirth management and medical monopoly: midwifery as (almost)

a profession. Journal of Nurse-Midwifery 29: 300–306.

Royal College of Midwives 2003 Valuing Practice: a Springboard for Midwifery Education. RCM, London.

Saunders D, Boulton M, Chapple J 2000 Evaluation of the Edgware Birth Centre. North Thames Perinatal Public Health, London.

Siddiqui J 1996 Midwifery values: part 1. British Journal of Midwifery 4(2): 87–89.

Stafford S 2001 Lack of autonomy: a reason for midwives leaving the profession? The Practising Midwife 4(7): 46–47.

Stein LI 1967 The Doctor–Nurse Game. Archives of General Psychology 16: 699–703.

Symon A 1994 Midwives and litigation 2: a small scale survey of attitudes. British Journal of Midwifery 2(4): 176–181.

Symonds I, Cullen L, Fraser D 2003 Evaluation of a formative inter-professional team objective structured clinical examination (ITOSCE): a method of shared learning in maternity education. Medical Teacher 25(1): 34–37.

Tew M 1990 Safer Childbirth? A Critical History of Maternity Care. Chapman & Hall, London.

Towler J, Bramall J 1986 Midwives in History and Society. Croom Helm, London.

Tyler S 1996 Independent midwives insurance: the stance of the RCM. British Journal of Midwifery 4(3): 151–152.

Further Reading

Marshall JE, Kirkwood S 2000 Autonomy and teamwork. In: Fraser D (ed), Professional Studies for Midwifery Practice. Churchill Livingstone, Edinburgh, pp. 127–141.
Discusses the role of the midwife as an autonomous practitioner in decision making by empowering women to make informed choices whilst working in collaboration with other members of the multidisciplinary team.

Nursing and Midwifery Council 2004a Midwives Rules and Standards. NMC, London.
All midwives should be familiar with the content of this publication, which clearly defines their statutory role and responsibilities and offers guidance and support in making autonomous decisions when caring for the childbearing woman and her baby.

Royal College of Midwives 1997 Debating Midwifery: Normality in Midwifery. RCM, London.
Publication that examines the concept of normality in relation to the statutory framework, research-based practice and the role of the midwife when planning and delivering maternity care to low-risk women.

Stein LI 1967 The Doctor–Nurse Game. Archives of General Psychology 16: 699–703.
Useful source should the midwife wish to further consider the interaction styles included in this chapter and compare with their own experiences of decision making in situations when medical colleagues have been involved.

Chapter 2

The Role of Knowledge in Midwifery Decision Making

Jeanne Siddiqui

INTRODUCTION: A PHILOSOPHICAL EXPLORATION

Whether professional decision making is based upon knowledge gathered from research, experience, theory or is simply described as 'gut-feeling' or intuition, it is the aim in this chapter to try and explain the way people *know* and to learn how they can use their knowledge in midwifery decision making.

It is acknowledged (Proctor and Renfrew 2000) that decision making in midwifery practice is influenced by a number of factors, and that the student may be *"confused by the apparent chaos of midwifery and its diffuse components"* (Clarke 2002: 84). Therefore, in order to determine what aspects of midwifery decision making can be consciously identified, explored and refined it is essential to sift through the perceived confusion of what constitutes midwifery knowledge.

The acquisition of knowledge and the nature of knowledge has provoked major philosophical debate for centuries. **Epistemology** – the study of knowledge – is a branch of philosophy that examines abstract theories about the concepts of knowledge, and from a midwifery point of view it is essential to examine what midwives *know* about childbirth and women in order to have an agreed and shared construct or representation of social reality about this very important event in human living.

THE IMPORTANCE OF KNOWLEDGE

It is reported (Plato ca. 428–ca. 348 BC) that the great philosopher, Socrates (470–399 BC) was, according to the Delphic Oracle, the wisest living person. Socrates interpreted this to mean that he was the wisest because he realised and admitted his own ignorance. It is also interesting to note that Socrates conducted his search for knowledge and therefore truth through a method of dialogue he called *'intellectual midwifery'* (Stumpf 1993: 36).

The search for knowledge or learning about the world we live in is a vital component of being human. It is also an obligation for midwives to identify a midwifery **body of knowledge** if they wish to be considered professional in the true sense of the word.

Midwifery knowledge comprises of many parts: theory (biology, physiology, psychology, sociology, historical, etc.), practice, research and perhaps most importantly, philosophy (what each individual midwife believes midwifery to be). If these component parts are not equally represented during midwifery education and training and valued in a philosophy for midwifery, then ultimately, the experience for women and the professional will be sub-optimal.

Imagine trying to help a woman and her baby breast feed without the underlying knowledge of physiology, without the experience of facilitating successful breastfeeding and the knowledge of psychological theories, without the foresight of well-conducted research, and without the sagacity of philosophical reasoning. The Royal College of Midwives (RCM 1991) found that women and babies were being subjected to dictatorial uneducated theories about breastfeeding and *". . . for a variety of reasons there was very little consistency between breastfeeding policies in different parts of the country and also between policy and practice within many individual institutions"* (RCM 1991, preface: page v). Such inconsistencies may continue to infiltrate the practice of modern midwives whose knowledge is incomplete. Although the example of breastfeeding is used, it may be that more areas of practice are affected due to a lack of knowledge that is not simply theoretical in nature.

WAYS OF KNOWING – HOW DO WE ACQUIRE KNOWLEDGE?

This question is at the centre of philosophical debate. Concepts are an idea or mental representation of what is understood or known, but how do individuals gain these concepts? Philosophers through the ages have considered the notion of 'God' and questioned how the idea or concept can be so universally accepted without people seeing 'God'. Hospers (1967) asks if it is possible that such a concept could be innate? Is it possible to understand or *know* something without having ever experienced it? The question could be asked of a midwife or doctor who has never given birth. Can they really *know* what it is like to have a baby?

This idea that something can be known without experiencing it is termed *Concept Rationalism* and is in direct opposition to the modern philosophical view of *Concept Empiricism,* which postulates that concepts are in some way derived directly from personal experiences in the world. According to this theory, individuals initially experience the physical world through the external senses of sight, touch, taste, smell and hearing. These first impressions are internalised by the brain and converted or recalled by the inner senses as feelings of pain, love, pleasure, etc. The relationship between the experience and the concept that is derived from it is highly subjective and personal and Hospers (1967: 111) considers that *". . . whatever the connection is between the concept and the experience, it is sufficiently indirect that no-one has given a clear account of exactly what this condition is in every case"*.

The philosopher John Locke (1632–1704) concluded that all **concepts** are derived from experience of the world. He divided the process of **concept** formation into two categories, the first category he called *ideas of sensation* and the second, *ideas of reflection* (Locke 1984). David Hume (1711–1776) carried this further by making the distinction between 'idea' and 'impression'. He theorised that there are no ideas without impressions. A person must first have the *impression* (the sense experience) in order to have the idea (Hume 1962). However, Hospers (1967, 1990) considered this rationale to be too simplistic and supported Locke's reasoning that there are *simple* and *complex* ideas – that it is possible to have an idea without actually experiencing or seeing something. There are many examples that demonstrate the combining of previous experiences or ideas to form new concepts (such as a golden mountain, a black rose – having probably seen a mountain and the colour gold separately and a rose and the colour black). However, Locke (1984) suggests that the human mind cannot create a single simple idea. If a person has never seen red, he or she cannot imagine it; similarly, if someone has never felt pain, they will not be able to imagine pain. This transference of simple to complex ideas is compared to the relationship of atoms to molecules.

"Without atoms, you cannot have molecules; and atoms can be combined in different ways to form different molecules. Without simple ideas, you cannot form complex ideas; but once you have a number of simple ideas, you can combine them in your imagination in all sorts of different ways to form the ideas of countless things that never existed on land or sea" (Hospers 1967: 104).

✎ Activity 2.1

With a partner, discuss the concept of 'green' and how this could be conveyed to a person who has been blind from birth. Note how difficult it is to do this without the simple concept of colour.

(Adapted from Hospers 1967)

✎ Activity 2.2

With a partner show how it is possible to build upon simple concepts by describing the following:

a) a unicorn
b) sadness
c) a lemon

(Adapted from Hospers 1967)

If simple concepts are connected to other ideas giving rise to even greater complex concepts (such as the concepts of black and roses to provide a concept or idea of a *black rose*), then one might assume that in order to develop a concept of childbirth without actually giving birth, a combination of concepts – pain, theoretical knowledge and observation – are used. It is also reasonable to assume that once a person has had a *direct experience* they then understand the concepts involved in that experience. This however, cannot always be substantiated as experience itself depends upon perception and the individuals' ability to express that perception in language that has the same meaning to others. For example, a woman experiencing childbirth may perceive it very differently from another woman who may be experiencing the same physiological process. The observer (midwife, doctor, birth partner) may see a process occurring and draw conclusions from it that then enables him or her to say they have a 'concept' of labour. Yet if it was so easy, there would be no difficulty in advising women what to expect in the process of labour. However, the most commonly expressed emotion from women following childbirth is that no-one told them what it was 'really like', a statement substantiated by Bradley et al. (1983) who highlighted discrepancies between midwives and women's perception of labour, and later by Baker et al. (2001).

This difficulty to define the concept of childbirth has had significant impact on the way that labour is managed, and led doctors in particular to **rationalise** the **concept**, to make it understandable and, more importantly, to control it. This led to protocols concerned with actively managing the process of labour, the differentiation and duration of the stages of labour and the increase in medical intervention in the process (O'Driscoll et al. 1975). Siddiqui (1992: 6) suggested that because:

". . . the concept of childbirth is indefinable in the experiential sense, it is therefore deemed unscientific so that if it is to be made sense of to those with a scientific background i.e. doctors, it must be confined within measurable limits".

The advent of epidural analgesia and more sophisticated pharmacological medications have removed much pain and suffering from childbirth, yet there can be a lack of understanding and even disbelief when women who have experienced a 'pain free' labour complain of dissatisfaction or feel unfulfilled because of this. The experience of childbirth is an *abstraction*. The semantic meaning of the word 'labour' denotes hard work, and whilst childbirth is surely this the word labour is too simplistic to completely portray the full meaning of the experience for each individual woman. Over a decade ago it was noted that: *"The act of childbirth has no adjective which can perfectly describe the feelings and emotions which occur in each individual woman at the time she experiences it"* (Siddiqui 1992: 6), and despite extensive research and theorizing related to communication in midwifery by McIntosh (1988), Kirkham (1993) and others (Tennant and Butler 1999), the concept remains as abstract as ever.

Activity 2.3

Write down what your concept (idea) of labour is. Think about how you have gained this concept, does it include:

a) Direct experience?
b) Observing women during labour?
c) Reading about childbirth?

Activity 2.4

Ask three women to describe their experiences of labour. Note the language they use (are they using simple concepts or complex ones?). In particular, ask them how they would pass on their understanding of the experience to others (their children, their friends, etc.).

THE NATURE OF MIDWIFERY KNOWLEDGE

In any exploration of what constitutes knowledge, the philosopher examines the acquisition and foundation of concepts. In historical, sociological and academic texts, it has been noted that numerous factors contribute to the existing **paradigms** of midwifery practice (Achterberg 1990, Riska and Wegar 1993, Tew 1990, Witz 1992). These texts and others supported midwifery research (Siddiqui 1992) where it was noted that:

- midwifery is complex and reliant upon sense-experience and perception;
- understanding of childbirth is impeded by imperfect and restrictive language used to express the meaning of abstract concepts;
- effective midwifery is reliant upon the relationship of the woman and the midwife;
- the proximity of midwifery to medicine cannot be overlooked;
- medical values and the traditional model of care employed by doctors has impacted significantly upon the current philosophy of midwifery.

Modern midwives rely upon knowledge gained through established theories, research, experience, problem-solving and sometimes *intuition* or tacit knowledge (the latter will be discussed in detail later). What is clear is that midwives examine questions that are conceptual abstractions that cannot be simply answered, observed or described. These questions are related to the nature of pain in childbirth, the emotional state of women during labour, the therapeutic relationship between mother and midwife during labour and many other abstract concepts. There have been difficulties in attempting to gain recognition of knowledge about these abstractions (Polyani 1962), because although logic may be the basis of this knowledge, analysis and explanation of it is often problematic because of the restrictions of language.

PHILOSOPHICAL ANALYSIS AND THE LANGUAGE OF MIDWIFERY

In philosophical exploration, the role of logical analysis is vital. Hospers (1967) gives the example of the statement 'all black cats are black' to show how the analytic properties of the statement can be demonstrated. There is a logical predicate of the sentence and it can be said to be 'true' without need for further investigation. To disagree and say that, 'all black cats are not black' would be to assert and deny the proposition and this would be a *contradiction*. This 'Law of Contradiction' (Kant 1790) was used to establish the truth of all *a priori* knowledge. However, the analytic quality of some propositions is not at all obvious or explicit. The statement 'all mothers have the best babies' is contradictory in nature, but when analysing what is meant by the word 'best', it may be seen that the subjective use of language influences understanding and meaning. The definitions of the statement are unclear and the proposition cannot be proved or disproved.

The problem with language is one of the fundamental challenges in philosophical argument and in knowledge acquisition. It may be concluded therefore, that most knowledge is general – that is, all mothers have babies. Sense experience on the other hand is particular – each mother's baby is the 'best' to her. Throughout the analytic process, the logicality and reliability of the method may be particularly influenced by the language used to describe the experience. Wittgenstein (1953) repeatedly counselled that language does not stand alone, it is intelligible only within the context in which it is used and how it is viewed by individuals making sense of the world around them. This is an important point when examining midwifery practice that has moved away from the social setting of the community into the institutional hierarchical setting of hospital with its dominant ideology of pathology.

Not only is it important to understand how language can restrict the ability to describe the world in which midwifery functions, it can also alienate midwives from the women they care for. Coded or euphemistic language used by midwives, not only perpetuates an aura of mystique about midwifery, but may contribute towards a perception of elitism or closure of ranks when things go wrong. The importance of the use of language in midwifery is that it may

reflect the philosophy of midwifery itself and be perceived as inclusive or conversely, may be seen to exclude the woman being cared for, creating barriers in the decision-making process.

✎ Activity 2.5

Consider the following language used between midwives to describe:

Full dilatation of the cervix; "*Mrs . . . is fully*".

A baby with a low Apgar score; "*The baby is flat*"

Now try to logically prove that the two statements are *true*

How inclusive is this language? If the woman hears the midwife saying these statements, would she understand them?

In summary, the context in which words are used to describe thoughts and feelings or knowledge and understanding is important when attempting to make sense of a complex life event such as childbirth. The essence or nature of midwifery is linked to indefinable concepts that often defy rationalist explanation from any other than a subjective perspective. Finally, the forming of concepts that contribute to midwifery knowledge must be examined in view of the factors that influence the individuals' experience (both midwife and woman) of the world. These concepts are related to the perception of the individual and the ability to express or communicate the experience to others in a language that has the same meaning for all.

TYPES OF KNOWLEDGE

Knowledge is acquired from a multitude of sources, and it is necessary to briefly examine the historical background of some of these so that the influences of midwifery knowledge and decision making may be identified

SCIENTIFIC KNOWLEDGE

The concept of 'science' first developed in Western Europe during a two-hundred-year period (1600–1800) known as the 'Age of Reason' or the 'Enlightenment' (Stumpf 1993) when there was a major change in human thinking. During this time there was an increasing faith in logical reasoning and an acceptance that individuals could influence the material world in which they lived. Humans were seen to 'progress' from one generation to the next and the belief in religious doctrine and authority was questioned and challenged.

The development of science and the resulting technological advances led to a change in world view that became known as **positivism**. This **positivistic** philosophy is difficult to define as it has had many different usages and interpretation over time. Originally introduced by Comte (1865), it was proposed to change the negative thinking of past philosophers and scientists by adopting a more *positive* approach to philosophic thinking, one that could provide all the answers to the knowledge that individuals seek in order to understand the world. One of the fundamental principles of **positivism** is that there is a common 'scientific method' to be used in the process of gaining knowledge. This scientific method, known as **induction** subjects all elements, including human sciences to a logical process of reduction whereby something is meaningful only if it can be observed through the senses. In other words 'seeing is believing'.

The **positivist** philosophy – later called scientific **empiricism** – has attracted many critics throughout the years (Kuhn 1962, Popper 1968); however, despite the decline of philosophical **positivism**, the role of **empirical** science remains the major contributor in the search for knowledge.

PERSONAL KNOWLEDGE AND EXPERIENCE

Whilst objecting to the view that science is able to provide all the answers required by human beings, the German philosopher Jürgen Habermas (1968) saw its place in the generation of knowledge, and his theory on *Knowledge and Human Interests* first published in 1968 may provide a useful framework for midwifery knowledge. Habermas (1987) proposed that the **empirical**-analytic sciences incorporate a *technical* element in the development of **cognitive** interest. In midwifery practice, the element of technical expertise is very apparent, and it would be foolhardy to reject the idea that a large amount of knowledge is gained from experiencing and observing midwifery practice (**empirical** evidence) in order to gain *technical* mastery. However, Habermas along with other philosophers such as Husserl (1859–1938), Heidegger (1889–1976) and Sartre (1905–1980) pursued other avenues of philosophical thought more concerned with understanding the nature of humanity within the world rather than simply expecting the natural world to provide all the answers through logical **empiricism**. What was later to become the development of **phenomenology** was described as ". . . *a different way of looking at philosophical problems such as the concept of the self, freewill, one's body, perception, values, language and metaphysics*" (Gray and Pratt 1991: 19).

Henry (1986) considered the phenomenological approach to be a compromise between the **rationalist** argument and the scientific approach to knowledge acquisition. The emphasis is placed upon the individual perspective and meaning of the situation for that person. Kant (1790), in his exploration of transcendental experience, concluded that having an experience itself does not provide clear meaning for the individual, it requires the individual to reflect upon the self-formative process of knowledge acquisition and to identify how knowledge through experience becomes personalised. This introduces another dimension into the process of knowledge acquisition, that of meaning *for us* along with meaning *in itself*.

When concepts are acquired in this way, the past experience guides the action and allows for a rapid perceptual grasp of the situation. This way of learning or acquiring knowledge has been expressed in a number of ways in nursing and midwifery curricula; by Jarvis (1992), Gibbs (1988) and Schön (1983, 1987) amongst others, who highlight the importance of making sense of experience within the context of everyday practice.

The main component of any learning from experience is establishing the *paradigm* – understanding that 'this is the way it is' or 'this is the way it works'. More importantly, the midwife who realises that **paradigms** can *shift* or change is learning that knowledge can change with experience and she must always be prepared to adapt to that change or alter the **paradigm**. Examples of **paradigmatic** shifting are experienced daily by student midwives. For example, students learn about post-partum haemorrhage in the classroom and observe the condition in practice. However, it is not until they actually deal with and put into practice all that they have learned, both theoretically and vicariously, that they realise they have established their own **paradigms** (knowing how 'it is' for them and how they dealt with it) and what adjustments they would make for future practice. Figure 2.1 illustrates this **paradigmatic** learning experience.

Decisions taken in midwifery practice hinge upon the midwife establishing **paradigms** – knowing how and knowing why. If actions are carried out only as part of a routine or task without considering the underpinning **paradigm**, the midwife cannot safely make decisions. To illustrate the above points, the example of orchestrated pushing is useful (see Activity 2.6). In the past, women were discouraged from spontaneous pushing during labour and only allowed to push under instruction from the midwife.

Activity 2.6

In the context of directed pushing during the second stage of labour, what sort of knowledge is the midwife utilising when deciding to practise in this way? Is practice based upon:

a) the midwife's paradigm?
b) an obstetric protocol?
c) current research?
d) routine practice?

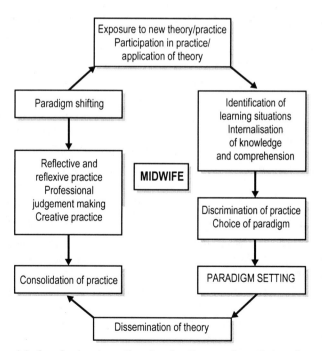

Figure 2.1   Adaptive model of professional practice showing the paradigmatic learning experience.

INTUITIVE KNOWLEDGE

Within the model (Figure 2.1), the idea of creative practice and judgement making is crucial, and is by no means based purely on **empirical** (sense experience) knowledge. Polyani (1962), Carper (1978) and Schön (1983), amongst others, have discussed knowledge gained through creative practice, through perceptive understandings of the nature of caring and formed the theory of **Praxis** – whereby the individual is able to reason and critically analyse the situation and most importantly is self-reflective. In this way, the individual can exert some control in his or her life, is able to manipulate objects and eventually creates new knowledge. According to Anderson et al. (1986), **praxis** reflects the **cognitive** aspects of the person. This ability leads caring professionals to list intuitive or **tacit** knowledge as an important element in their repertoire of skills. Silva (1977 in Gray and Pratt, 1991: 5) endorsed this view:

> *"The time has come to value truths arrived at by intuition and introspection as much as those arrived at by scientific experimentation".*

Midwifery is multi-faceted and the concept of intuition raises questions about how midwives explain this way of 'knowing'. During midwifery research (Siddiqui 1995), one midwife tried to explain it in the following way:

> *"It might be something in the rapport we have with women . . . it's empathy, it's not easy to gain that sort of experience, you need to be very receptive. Midwives are usually very receptive and open". [transcript 112].*

This view was expressed by many midwives who pursued this notion of an *"awareness creating relationship"* (Kirby 1990) that goes beyond the administering of clinical procedures and processes. Midwives talked about 'keying in' to the situation, and being 'in tune' with women. Interestingly, doctors who were asked about this aspect of knowledge felt less comfortable with leaving the exploration in abstract terms, and rationalised the concept

in relation to experience gained previously and stored subconsciously for utilisation at a later date.

Linked to this aesthetic ability to create a knowledge of the world of women during childbirth through receptiveness and perceptive communications, midwives are also charged with the inherent task of empowering those they care for, enabling women to make decisions about their care based on individual needs (Rule 6, NMC 2004). Using the principles of Habermas' (1968) theory of a philosophical model, the element of *emancipatory freedom* is useful when considering the empowerment of women. Habermas (1968) maintains that all knowledge is gained in the pursuit of **cognitive** interests which can be: *technical* – where the natural sciences seek to assert technical mastery over nature; *hermeneutic* – seeking to further understand human beings by interpreting their purposes, motives and intentions (originally this was through the analysis of written historical texts) through their actions; and *emancipatory* – seeking freedom from constraint, particularly from distorted communications of ideology which claim that **empirical**-analytic knowledge is the *only* form of legitimate knowledge.

By developing a practical attitude, that balances the technical, hermeneutic and emancipatory interests, an *"action-orienting culture"*(Habermas 1968: 307) develops where there is mutual respect of other professions and a sharing of knowledge, together with the potential intent of empowering the client. According to Kirby and Slevin (1992: 75):

> *"Empowerment is care realised. It is the liberation of the persons so that they have freedom to realise their potential with dignity and in a personal responsible way".*

Therefore, the midwife, by creating a bond of understanding between herself and the client should be enabled to function at a high level of thinking due to the *dispositional state* she willingly places herself in through the nature of the caring process. With this element of the person being central to the process a unique therapeutic relationship is fostered, one identified by midwives as being 'in tune' or 'keying in' to the situation. Vincent (1993), in her work with lay birth attendants in Indonesia, identified this relationship between the midwife and her client as a spiritual experience where the midwife was afforded a *'spiritual mandate'* during this intimate period. She describes how the spiritual aspect of midwifery was manifested both in the way in which the midwife receives this spiritual power and in the use of it in her work as an 'authoritative' source of knowledge:

"I see it as a form of authoritative knowledge; but of a kind that is hidden far more profoundly than the knowledge of modern doctors as only someone who has been touched by the spirit has access to it. To the modern world, this makes it extremely suspect, as the knowledge is only available when it is needed". (Vincent 1993: 10).

In westernised countries such as Britain, there is no recognised 'spiritual mandate' for midwives. However, the recommendation from successive governments (DoH 1992, 1993) for midwives to provide continuity of care and the need to provide 'holistic' care, indicates a subliminal expectation from society that a certain sensitivity is required, and a growing acknowledgement that the relationship between the woman and the midwife is important in ensuring a successful outcome.

In terms of knowledge acquisition, it may be that this relationship between the woman and her midwife is the key component of midwifery knowledge, unique from any other form of professional knowledge, allowing the development of an awareness-creating relationship that is the foundation of midwifery practice.

AUTHORITATIVE KNOWLEDGE AND KNOWLEDGE AS POWER

In healthcare, the person's right to be autonomous is often compromised by a lack of knowledge or information that is needed to make an informed decision (see Chapter 1). Whilst personal autonomy is seen to be morally desirable, the issue of professional autonomy is

a particular concern in midwifery. By implication, without professional autonomy, the ability to empower clients in the decision-making process is impossible (see Chapter 9). Recent emphasis on quality and effectiveness in clinical practice, together with the introduction of Clinical Governance (DoH 1997) has somewhat diminished the autonomy of doctors, demanding more accountability and transparency. However, medicine remains a powerful force within society as a whole (Friedson 1976, Witz 1992), with medical knowledge seen as superior to other professions (Fryer 1992, Siddiqui 1995). When medical knowledge is held to be superior to any other form of knowledge in the provision of maternity care, it is logical to assume that decisions regarding how care is delivered will be based upon that knowledge, hence the predominance of an obstetric philosophy and approach to care that favours intervention, manipulation and control. Only by continuing education and by challenging the myth of medical superiority can midwives hope to influence midwifery care in the future. Tew (1990: 10) reminds midwives of the power of using a philosophy that is in harmony with the ethos of the profession:

"If the traditional model of midwifery, that of 'masterly inactivity' and the premise that childbirth is a normal physiological event still existed, the midwife would have no difficulty in acting as advocate for the autonomy of the mother. The mothers' right to self-determination would be absolute".

Midwives themselves may perpetuate the belief that they are subservient to or less powerful than doctors, perceiving themselves to be of a lower professional status (Siddiqui 1995). Interestingly, doctors do not always share this perception:

"I think midwives are at a level just below consultants. They get a good grounding in midwifery and have a moderate understanding of medicine, their knowledge of obstetrics is good but it is the technical skills of obstetrics which they do not have". (Siddiqui 1995: transcript 116 – obstetrician).

The strength of decision making in midwifery therefore relies upon the midwife being confident in his or her knowledge, not only of obstetric theory, but also in the constituents of the relationship between the midwife and the woman. This relationship must be confidently promoted to be the foundation of a unique source of knowledge, inherent in a philosophy that is consistently demonstrated by midwives in practice. Based upon respect for persons and including the major ethical principles of autonomy, beneficence, non-maleficence and justice (see Chapter 7).

KNOWLEDGE ACQUIRED THROUGH RESEARCH AND EVIDENCE-BASED PRACTICE

Decision making in midwifery can only be effective if it is based upon knowledge that is *informed*, that is aware of all the current theories. During the past decade there has been an explosion of knowledge, not only in terms of the amount of research undertaken and subsequent theories that have been generated, but also in respect of the sources available from which to retrieve information. The skill needed to conduct a thorough search of all information sources is one that midwives need to acquire (Stanton and Fraser 2000). If no other professional updating is undertaken but this one, then a great deal will have been achieved.

Midwives also need to think carefully before embarking upon small-scale research projects by asking themselves 'so what?'. Will a project add to the body of midwifery knowledge? Is it ethically acceptable to capitalise upon a vulnerable conveniently accessible population of pregnant women just to undertake a study for educational purposes? Many degree theses are not disseminated or exposed to the scrutiny of peer review. These aspects are key concerns in the expansion of midwifery knowledge and should be considered when deciding upon a research topic.

The philosophical foundations of research should be considered so that the methods chosen reflect the researcher's particular orientation toward his or her view of the world. Bryman (2001: 4) states:

"Methods are not simply neutral tools; they are linked with the ways in which the researcher or social scientist makes the connection between different viewpoints about the nature of social reality".

If midwives wish to represent the world as it is experienced by pregnant women or by other midwives, it is important to do this using predominantly *qualitative* methods, the purpose of which is to seek meaning and enhance understanding. Experimental or quantitative methods should be used only where absolutely necessary, and where cause and effect are the main aims. Researchers should be able to rationalise and defend methodologies with the main component being transferability into the clinical situation. Measuring outcomes in statistical rather than human terms ought to be the exception rather than the rule in midwifery research.

Henry and Pashley (1990) proposed that central to qualitative enquiry is the **phenomenological** idea of how the individual person interacts in a world of everyday commonsense experience. This (**phenomenological**) approach attempts to explore the meaning of experience through understanding the person's own perception and interpretation of the experience. Once midwives admit that a major source of midwifery knowledge is based upon sense perception and experience, the conclusions that can be drawn from future experiences will be arrived at through **deductive** reasoning rather than **inductive** (theory generated) approaches.

✎ Activity 2.7

Consider the *truth* of the following statements:

The mother is experiencing painful uterine contractions;

Contractions are necessary in order to expel the fetus;

Therefore the woman is in labour.

The premise (first statement) in Activity 2.7 is an occurrent state, experienced by the mother, whilst the inference (second statement) is based upon the midwife's experience. The conclusion (third statement) would have been arrived at using knowledge gained through experience, not only of the external sense perception but equally through the internal senses and the dispositional state of the midwife. The midwife's knowledge, together with the mother's behaviour, physical position, breathing pattern and the reported pain perceptions leads the midwife to the conclusion through the process of **deductive** reasoning.

If the same scenario was examined using the **empirical** 'scientific' criteria necessary for **inductive** theory, the conclusion may be different with serious implications for the mother and fetus (see Activity 2.8):

✎ Activity 2.8

Consider the *truth* of the following statements:

The mother is experiencing painful uterine contractions

Contractions must be accompanied by cervical dilatation

If cervical dilatation is not occurring, the mother is not in labour

---

This is a well-known obstetric viewpoint (O'Driscoll et al. 1975), and has influenced the decisions taken by obstetricians and midwives regarding the management of labour for nearly three decades. Because the expected **empirical** criteria is not met, the woman may be diagnosed as 'not in labour'. The argument may be *valid* but this does not necessarily mean it is *true*. The conclusion follows logically from the premises but is *invalid* because **phenomenological** data such as time, space and perception are not incorporated into the statements. Whilst it may be true that <u>eventually</u> the cervix must dilate, the occurrent state of labour without cervical dilatation may also be true.

By conducting practice based on theory derived through one type of research alone (experimental/quantitative), the understanding of the experience is limited or reduced to the mechanical aspects only. By undertaking qualitative research into midwifery, a balanced and rounded view can be obtained. Similarly when reviewing research, it is important to look for studies that not only consider the cause and effect of a particular situation or condition but those that attempt to explain the meaning or interpret the experience from the view of the participant.

SUMMARY AND CONCLUSION

In order to understand what influences midwifery decision-making, it is necessary to explore the sources of midwifery knowledge so that there is an agreed and shared idea (construct) of social reality about what midwifery *is*. Different ways of knowing influence midwifery, and it is important to acknowledge intuitive or tacit knowledge and the role it plays in making clinical decisions alongside theoretical, scientific and historical knowledge. At the same time, midwives should recognise that science cannot exclusively describe social reality and if all knowledge sources are not equally represented and valued within a philosophy for midwifery, then ultimately, decision-making will be biased towards one or the other and the experience for women and the professional will be sub-optimal.

The core of any knowledge is the *concept* or simple idea; from this other ideas and concepts may develop. If, however, the simple concept is indefinable, as it is in childbirth, then decisions made by doctors and midwives may be based upon distorted constructs and concepts. Because the nature of midwifery knowledge is so complex, it requires midwives to conceptualise at a high level of abstract thinking, being able to understand not only the scientific elements of knowledge but also to comprehend the structure and function of language as both a means and a limitation of communication. Midwives must also be able to recognise when an established paradigm has 'shifted' to make way for a different way of 'knowing'. Being confident in a body of professional knowledge that is midwifery should allow midwives to demonstrate a commitment to a philosophy of practice that is woman centred. This should be based upon respect for persons and ethics, and is developed through an appreciation of the role of appropriate research so that midwives can be discriminatory in deciding what is necessary for contemporary practice.

KEY POINTS FOR BEST PRACTICE

- It is necessary for the midwife to continuously reflect upon what constitutes midwifery knowledge, how it has been acquired and how it is used in professional practice.

- The component parts of knowledge should be *equally* represented and valued during midwifery education, practice and research.

- It is essential that midwives identify and articulate when intuitive or tacit

knowledge informs their practice so that its value may be accounted for in the process and classification of evidence that contributes to the development of clinical guidelines such as those published by the National Institute of Clinical Excellence (see Chapter 3).

- The importance of the use of language in midwifery practice is that it should reflect the philosophy of midwifery itself and should not exclude women or create barriers in the decision–making process.

- Midwives who are able to reflect upon past professional experiences and use them to establish paradigms of practice are functioning at a high level of cognitive ability. It is through this development in knowledge acquisition that midwives may improve the care and ultimately clinical outcomes for both women and babies.

References

Achterberg J 1990 Woman as Healer. Rider, London.

Anderson RJ, Hughes JA, Sharrock WW 1986 Philosophy and the Human Sciences. Croom Helm, London.

Baker A, Ferguson SA, Roach GD, Dawson D 2001 Perceptions of labour pain by mothers and their attending midwives. Journal of Advanced Nursing 35(2): 171–179.

Bradley C, Brewin CR, Duncan SLB 1983 Perceptions of labour: discrepancies between midwives' and patients' ratings. British Journal of Obstetrics and Gynaecology 90(12): 1176–1179.

Bryman A 2001 Social Research Methods. Oxford University Press, Oxford.

Carper BA 1978 Fundamental Patterns of Knowing in Nursing. Advances in Nursing Science 1: 13–23.

Clarke H 2002 A Personal Philosophy of Midwifery. British Journal of Midwifery 10(2): 84–87.

Comte A 1865 A General View of Positivism. In: Stumpf SE (1993) Socrates to Sartre: A History of Philosophy Fifth Edition. McGraw-Hill, New York.

Department of Health 1992 Health Committee Second Report on Maternity Services (Chair: Nicholas Winterton). HMSO, London.

Department of Health 1993 Changing Childbirth: Report of the Expert Maternity Group (Chair: Baroness Cumberlege); Part I. HMSO, London.

Department of Health 1997 The New NHS: Modern-Dependable. DoH, London.

Friedson E 1976 Professional Powers: A Study of the Sociology of Applied Knowledge. Dodd, New York.

Fryer N 1992 Philosophical aspects within the midwifery curriculum. Journal of Advances in Health and Nursing Care 1(5): 61–83.

Gibbs G 1988 Learning by Doing: A Guide to Teaching and Learning Methods. EMU, Oxford.

Gray G, Pratt R 1991 Towards a Discipline of Nursing. Churchill Livingstone, Melbourne.

Habermas J 1968 Knowledge and Human Interests, trans. JJ Shapiro. Heinemann, London.

Heidegger M 1962 Being and Time. SCM Press, London.

Henry C 1986 The Concept of the Person. Unpublished PhD thesis, Leeds University.

Henry C, Pashley G 1990 Health and Nursing Studies for Diploma and Undergraduate Students: Health Ethics. Quay, Lancaster.

Hospers J 1967 An Introduction to Philosophical Analysis (Revised Edition). Routledge and Kegan Paul, London.

Hospers J 1990 An Introduction to Philosophical Analysis

(Third Edition). Routledge, London.

Hume D 1962 Dialogues Concerning Human Understanding. The Liberal Arts Press, New York.

Husserl E 1965 Phenomenology and the Crisis of Philosophy. Harper and Row, New York.

Jarvis P 1992 Reflective practice and nursing. Nurse Education Today 12: 174–181.

Kant I 1790 The critique of judgement. In: Anderson RJ, Hughes JA, Sharrock WW (eds) 1985 Philosophy and the Human Sciences. Croom Helm, London.

Kirby C 1990 Caring in a divided community (unpublished essay). In: Slevin O, Buckenham M (eds), 1992 Project 2000: The Teachers Speak. Campion Press, Edinburgh.

Kirby C, Slevin O 1992 A new curriculum of care. In: Slevin O, Buckenham M (eds), 1992, Project 2000: The Teachers Speak. Campion Press, Edinburgh.

Kirkham M 1993 Communication in midwifery. In: Alexander J, Levy V, Roch S (eds), Midwifery Practice. Macmillan, London.

Kuhn TS 1962 The Structure of Scientific Revolutions. University of Chicago Press, Chicago.

Locke J 1894 Essay Concerning Human Understanding. Dover Publications, New York. (2 volumes).

McIntosh J 1988 Women's views of communication in labour and delivery. Midwifery 4: 166.

Nursing and Midwifery Council 2004 Midwives Rules and Standards, Rule 6 Responsibilities and Sphere of Practice, p. 17, 2 August 2004. NMC, London.

O'Driscoll K, Carrroll C, Coughlan M 1975 Selective Induction of Labour. British Medical Journal 2: 727–729.

Plato (ca. 428–ca. 348 BC) The Last Days of Socrates, trans. H. Tredennick 1954, Penguin Classics.

Polyani M 1962 Personal Knowledge. Routledge and Kegan Paul, London.

Popper K 1968 The Logic of Scientific Discovery. Hutchinson, London.

Proctor S, Renfrew M (eds) 2000 Linking Research and Practice in Midwifery: A Guide to Evidence-Based Practice. Baillière Tindall, London. Introduction, p. 2.

Riska E, Wegar K (eds) 1993 Gender, Work and Medicine: Women and the Medical Division of Labour. Sage International Sociological Association, London.

Royal College of Midwives 1991 Successful Breastfeeding, 2nd edn. Churchill Livingstone, London.

Sartre JP 1976 The Critique of Dialectical Reason. NLB, London.

Schön D 1983 The Reflective Practitioner: How Professionals Think in Action. Temple Smith, London.

Schön D 1987 Educating the Reflective Practitioner. Jossey Bass, London.

Siddiqui J 1992 Midwifery: Science or Art? Journal of Advances in Health and Nursing Care 1(5): 3–12.

Siddiqui J 1995 Conceptions of Midwifery: A Study of Forms of Knowledge and Values Foundational for Midwifery Unpublished MPhil thesis, University of Central Lancashire.

Silva M 1977 Philosophy, science, theory: interrelationships and implications for nursing research. In: Nicoll LH (ed), 1986 Perspectives on Nursing Theory. Little Brown, Boston, pp. 563–568.

Stanton W, Fraser D 2000 Accessing the literature. In: Fraser D (ed), Professional Studies in Midwifery Practice. Churchill Livingstone, London, Chapter 1, pp. 1–21.

Stumpf SE 1993 Socrates to Sartre: A History of Philosophy, 5th edition. McGraw-Hill Inc., New York.

Tennant J, Butler M 1999 Communication: Issues for Change. British Journal of Midwifery 7(6): 359–362.

Tew M 1990 Safer Childbirth: A Critical History of Maternity Care. Chapman & Hall, London.

Vincent P 1993 When the Spirit Calls: Becoming a Midwife in a Traditional Society, Newsletter – Birth Traditions Survival Bank Centre for Learning, Agriculture and Appropriate Technology, P.O. Box 57 Kodaidanal 624101 Tamil-Nadu, India.

Wittgenstein L 1953 Philosophical Investigations. Blackwell, Oxford.

Witz A 1992 Professions and Patriarchy. The International Library of Sociology. Routledge, London.

Further Reading

Hospers J (1990) An Introduction to Philosophical Analysis, 3rd edition. Routledge, London, Chapter 1, pp. 32–51.

Chapter 3

Using the Evidence to Inform Decisions

Elizabeth R. Cluett

INTRODUCTION

Evidence-based practice (EBP) is advocated as a key component for quality midwifery practice, and indeed for all healthcare practice, being a core element in several government publications including Changing Childbirth (Department of Health [DoH] 1993), The New NHS (DoH 1997), A First Class Service (DoH 1998), and The NHS Plan (NHS Executive 2000). One of the lynch pins to a quality maternity service is therefore the decision making undertaken by individual midwives as well as those responsible for the organisation of maternity services at all levels, as to what is the best available evidence. The next decision is how can the evidence be used to ensure that maternity care facilitates women's choices, is delivered in a caring context, and is both clinically and cost effective. Clinical Governance is about ensuring excellence in practice (DoH 1999), and it could be argued that this is most likely to be achieved if all involved in healthcare make evidence-based decisions.

As EBP is fundamental to modern midwifery practice this chapter will explore what constitutes evidence and the relationship between evidence and research; how evidence can be identified, accessed, evaluated, interpreted and applied to practice; thus considering the meaning of evidence based midwifery practice and how evidence can be used to inform clinical decision making. Examples will be used to illustrate the interdependence of clinical skills, woman centred care and research data as evidence in the decision making processes for practice. Some research principles will be presented alongside discussion of EBP.

DEFINING EVIDENCE AND EVIDENCE-BASED PRACTICE

Evidence-based practice was originally called 'evidence-based medicine'. It is believed to have developed in association with 'problem-based learning', which was first described as an educational method by McMaster University in Canada (Evidence based medicine working group 1992), although Sackett et al. (2000) suggest earlier examples. **Problem-based learning** – also called 'enquiry-based learning' – is when students are helped to identify for themselves what they need to know to provide high-quality care, then enabled in the development of the skills to access the knowledge, and ultimately the competencies to practice EBP (Cleverley 2003, Price 2003). In practice, the concept is that healthcare decisions – and hence clinical care – are based directly on identifiable sources of evidence open to critical appraisal. These concerns are further explored in Chapter 6.

'Evidence' can be material, such as a placenta indicating a recent birth, but more often evidence is understood to be facts that testify to a particular event or situation. This implies that 'evidence' is information or knowledge about something. Evidence-based practice is therefore practice based on knowledge (see Chapter 2). Indeed, Proctor and Renfrew (2000) considered 'knowledge-based practice' in preference to evidence-based practice, because knowledge was perceived to be more encompassing of the multifaceted influences within midwifery. Understanding 'evidence' using this broad definition means that evidence includes personal experience from life and midwifery; traditional and professional knowledge, such as that handed on from experts; scientific and technological information, which may relate to the fields of psychology, sociology, physiology, information technology and many more; as well as research evidence.

Practice is not just doing what is known, it is about working with individuals, appreciating their perspective, assessing their needs and wishes, linking that to our knowledge, resources and abilities, and about generating new ideas, adapting them to the individual situation. Thus, practice is creative, innovative, sensitive as well as knowledge-based. So evidence-based practice is a philosophy of care, in which midwives, and all practitioners, strive to provide the very best care to each individual, utilising not only evidence but also their own creative, analytical and personal skills. Describing EBP as a philosophy could give the impression that it is a nebulous term – something for academics to debate – but actually nothing could be further from the truth. EBP is a practical way of working. It can be practised by the most experienced expert, and by the newest student, and most importantly the woman is central to/involved in the whole process. The key aim of EBP is to enable practitioners to make decisions about which is the best care option(s) for particular individuals or groups. The most-often cited definition for the decision-making process that is EBP is:

"The conscientious, explicit and judicious use of the current best evidence in making decisions about the care of individual patients." (Sackett et al. 1996: 71).

There are several things that EBP is not. First, it is not static; evidence is forever changing in the light of new research, new technology and new ideas, not to mention old ideas and options put together in a new way. Therefore, EBP must be viewed like every birth; the same process, but unique and new every time. This is a challenge as it means no one can establish what is the best practice, and set that information in guidelines once and for all, never to be updated. The onus is on each practitioner to establish the evidence for each case. However, the bonus is that it never gets dull, and there is always something to learn. Thus, the EBP midwife is a thinking, questioning, learning practitioner open to new ideas and ways of working.

Evidence-based practice can facilitate choice as it can provide information about each option; however, it has been argued that EBP can be restrictive (DaCruz 2002), limiting choice to practitioners and clients. Vaginal breech could be an example of this (Robinson 2001), and since Hannah et al. (2000) undertook their trial, vaginal breech births are rare. The choice here is limited by two factors. First, women are pressured into accepting elective Caesarean section (Robinson 2001), presumably because of the way in which the evidence is presented. Second, fewer practitioners have the skills to support women who would consider a vaginal breech birth, so women may not find a practitioner willing and competent to provide this option. However, it could be argued that it is not EBP that has limited choice here, but the way in which the research evidence has been used. While Hannah et al. (2000) provided strong evidence, there is an alternative research perspective. Albrecht et al. (2002) undertook a comparative prospective study and concluded that for women at low risk of complication, vaginal breech was a reasonable option. While this is not a randomised controlled trial (RCT), it is a reasonable study and if the perspective of the woman, her unique situation and wishes are considered, then the decision making based on all the 'evidence' may be very different. As Haynes (2002: 1350) stated, ". . . evidence does not make decisions, people do." The evidence is neutral – it is how the evidence is used that affects practice. Practitioners need to consider very carefully their decisions as to the types of evidence used to make practice decisions, including the weighting given to the various types of evidence, not only for each individual woman, but also for the wider maternity service and professional practice. Key to this is remembering the definition of evidence given at the start of this section. This is arguably the key difference between practice which is research-based and evidence-based. When 'research' was the criterion, there was the potential for other forms of evidence and the unique needs of the women to be overlooked, in the rigid implementation of the latest research. This is not evidence-based practice.

THE EVIDENCE-BASED PRACTICE PROCESS

The first and most crucial decision is to adopt an evidence-based approach and start looking at every aspect of practice with an enquiring mind. The EBP process can be described as a series of five steps (Sackett et al. 2000). The decision(s) made at each step affect the subsequent elements in the process, the steps being:

* Framing the question
* Finding all the evidence
* Appraising that evidence
* Applying the conclusions to the case
* Evaluating the outcomes, of the case and the process.

Undertaking the full EBP process steps is a time-consuming activity, and requires some skill. All midwives could undertake the process, although to date not all have had the education or resources to do so. Also, in the real world of maternity care, there is not time for everyone to conduct the full process for themselves for every case/scenario. Therefore, a modified EBP consists of the following steps:

* Framing the question
* Accessing literature that has been appraised and collated on the topic
* Applying the conclusions to practice
* Evaluating the outcomes, of the case and the process.

Appraised literature is usually national and/or local guidelines, and published systematic reviews, thus bypassing the critical appraisal of original data, which is the most intellectually demanding and time-consuming step within the process. The following sections will explore each of the steps in both the shortened and full EBP pathways, within the context of midwifery practice.

FRAMING THE QUESTION

The aim of EBP is to find answer(s) to clinical questions, and is the common starting point for both pathways. The source of questions can be very diverse, and include midwives, student midwives, women and their families and the general public. Reading midwifery and related literature should generate as many questions in the reader as it answers, and a similar response should occur to news and multimedia information. Practitioners and clients should be encouraged to ask 'why' and 'who said' to almost every aspect of care. Women may not always have the ability to articulate their questions, or may not know which questions need asking. Therefore, the midwife has a very important role in actively encouraging the woman's participation, either individually or as part of a group.

Just asking questions is not enough – they need to be well-structured questions. The questions that relate to the underpinning knowledge-based were called by Sackett et al. (2000) 'background questions'; they are topic-focused and may be based on the various '-ologies', for example:

* What causes pre-eclampsia?
* Why do women want children?
* How do families work?

Then there are the care-related questions, or the foreground questions (Sackett et al. 2000). These are client or client group-specific, action-orientated, and outcome-related. Some examples are provided in Box 3.1. Some of the questions have a comparative component.

Care-related questions can be about how issues/conditions are identified or diagnosed, how adverse events can be prevented, management options/choices, or about outcomes for women, their infants, the service or the professionals involved. The aim is that questions are as objective and specific as possible. Several questions to cover all the

required aspects are better than one long complex question. A neutral expectation should be adopted, akin to null hypotheses for experimental research (Cluett 2000) (see Box 3.2 for examples). The decisions made about how a question is framed determine what

---

Box 3.1 Examples of Care-Related Questions

1. Is labouring in water safe for women at low risk of complications?

Here, the *client group* is 'women at low risk of complications', the *action* is 'labouring in water', and the outcome is the safety, which could be maternal, fetal or hopefully both, and the *implied comparative group* is women not labouring in water.

2. Do Sure Start projects increase local breast feeding rates?

Here, the *implied client group* is women within a Sure Start catchment area, the *action* is the project and the *outcome* the breast feeding rate.

3. Can routine vaginal swabs identify all women who are colonised with Group B *Streptococcus*?

Here, the *client group* is all women with Group B *Streptococcus*, the *action* is the screening process, and the outcome is successful identification and prevention of neonatal infection.

Box 3.2 Neutral Questions for Evidence-Based Activity

* How does birthing in water affect perineal trauma?
  rather than
  Is perineal trauma reduced in waterbirths?
* What are the breast feeding rates within Sure Start areas?
  rather than
  Do Sure Start projects increase local breast feeding rates?

information is sought during the EBP process and ultimately used in practice.

SEARCHING FOR THE EVIDENCE

Once the question has been decided, the next step is to locate the evidence. The main sources of evidence are:

1. people, for example experts, ourselves, colleagues, students and women;
2. literature.

These can be linked with people guiding us to specific literature sources. There is a multitude of literature sources, and the quality of the evidence found in them can vary considerably. There are also many different types of literature. Therefore, the type and source of information used to answer a question is one of the most important decisions made in the EBP process.

TYPES OF LITERATURE

Literature can broadly be divided into either primary or secondary. Primary literature is original data, such as original research, case studies or audits. Secondary literature includes reviews, explanations, discussions, editorials, critiques, guidelines, opinions and letters. Literature may be published – as in books, journals, theses or government/trust reports – or unpublished – such as research data held by the researcher or personal knowledge from an expert.

The textbook is the most traditional source of evidence, the authors sharing their knowledge. It is possible to get a book published merely by having the money and determination to do so. The very best textbooks are multi-authored by experts, who have researched and evaluated all aspects of their topic, before presenting it in a well-referenced, up-to-date, chapter. This usually has to be within a prescribed number of words, understandable by wide readership, and still current 12 months later, which represents the minimum interval from writing to publication. So, textbooks have a role in providing background information which tends to change less frequently and be less client-specific, but are less helpful in answering most EBP questions.

Journals are the next source of information for most professionals. There are a variety of journals, from the profession-specific that aim to keep the reader up to date with topical issues and news, to those that collate and summarize the key research. What is published is likely to be affected by the overall aims of the journal, the readership, and the influence of its editors/board. The quality of the original research may be variable, depending on whether or not the material is peer reviewed (the process whereby submitted articles are critically appraised by experts in that field) before publication. The number of journals – not to mention their cost – prohibits even the most avid reader from accessing them all.

Online journals and associated services are very useful. *Midwifery Information and Resources Service* (MIDIRS), the *British Medical Journal* (BMJ) and *The Lancet*, to mention just a few, offer alert services for topics you have informed them are of particular interest to you. This is a great way of keeping generally up to date on the key areas of your practice, and is recommended to practitioners. Maternity services should facilitate access to such databases within the work setting. However, to answer a specific question, a search across all the databases and journals must be carried out. The first decision is whether to undertake a full EBP search to access the original data for review, or the shortened pathway, to identify and access pre-appraised literature. The choice will be affected by the expertise of the individual and the time scale. Both processes will be outlined.

ACCESSING PRE-APPRAISED LITERATURE: THE SHORT EBP PROCESS

Here, the aim is to access literature that has been identified and critically appraised by experts and then, if it is applicable, to base practice on that evidence. Pre-appraised literature includes guidelines, systematic reviews and meta-analyses.

(i) Guidelines

The first place to search is local clinical guidelines, which may be available through an intranet or as a written document. These guidelines should be produced by a multi-disciplinary team, reflect local needs, be up to date, evidence-based and well-referenced. Such guidelines are consistent with clinical governance (NHS Executive 1999). If there are not local evidence-based guidelines, then this needs addressing.

National guidelines are becoming increasingly available, such as electronic fetal monitoring by the National Institute for Clinical Excellence (NICE 2001), Anti D prophylaxis (NICE 2002), and antenatal care (NICE 2003a). There are also guidelines from professional organisations; for example, the Royal College of Midwives (RCM) positions statements on the use of water in labour and birth (RCM 2000) or home birth (RCM 2002). The Royal College of Obstetricians and Gynaecologists (RCOG) publishes Clinical Green Top Guidelines, for example Thromboembolic Disease in Pregnancy and the Puerperium: Acute Management (RCOG 2001).

Any guideline should be evaluated. This involves: checking who wrote the guideline, whether midwives and ideally consumers as well as any relevant medical staff; when it was last reviewed; the quality of the evidence on which it is based; and whether or not it is well-referenced. While interprofessional guidelines are ideal – and these should clearly have the woman at the centre of care – midwives should have midwifery guidelines. These need to be flexible and supportive (Rogers 2002).

(ii) Systematic Reviews and Meta-Analyses

A **systematic review** is when all the available data, both published and unpublished, on a particular topic is collated and then critically appraised to enable conclusion for best practice to be drawn in the light of the available data and its quality. This is a detailed and logical process that needs to be clearly articulated as part of the review; in this way the readers can decide if the conclusions presented are based on an open evaluation of all the information available. Systematic reviews should include all the available evidence on a topic. This includes data from experimental and non-experimental research, as well as descriptive and comparative data that may have been collected for original research or as part of maternity data. At present, most of the data are quantitative in nature.

A specific type of systematic review is the **meta-analysis**. This is where the available data accessed and reviewed and statistical analysis is conducted to combine to produce results from the various sources, recognising any particular strengths or weaknesses in the original papers. Undertaking systematic reviews at this level is a research process in its own right.

Systematic reviews are published in Evidence-Based Journals for medicine, nursing and several specialities. The published reviews are usually on topical issues, often associated with new research papers that provide new/updated evidence. These papers vary from very detailed reviews, to updates and summaries. The Royal College of Midwives published its own journal *Evidence Based Midwifery* in June 2003. The first edition contained peer-reviewed original research, rather than systematic reviews, so arguably this is a research journal rather than an evidence-based one.

For midwives, a key source of systematic reviews is the Cochrane Library. Teams of practitioners – often including several professionals and increasingly involving a consumer – review topics and take responsibility for ensuring that the reviews are updated. There are very clear guidelines as to the criteria used for literature searches and reviews, which are published with the review. The Cochrane Library is a vital resource for all midwives, and practitioners should ensure that they access the data. Access can usually be via local health service libraries, and is increasingly through web facilities in the work place. Another very useful resource for reviews is the Centre for Reviews and Dissemination (CRD); this was established in 1994, under the auspices of the University of York, and has reviews on most healthcare-related topics. Its aim is to promote evidence-based practice across the NHS (www.york.ac.uk/inst/crd).

Systematic reviews/meta analyses utilise quantitative data, and although accompanied with an explanatory text, an understanding of the basics of data analysis is required. The most common statistical terms used are odds ratios (OR), numbers needed to treat (NNT), relative risk (RR), *p*-values and confidence intervals (CI). Midwives need to undertake research awareness/appreciation education.

Having accessed the pre-appraised literature, you must ensure that it does answer your question, is applicable to your/the client's circumstances, and that it is suggesting options which are available locally. If there is any doubt about the usefulness/applicability of the evidence, it is advisable to consult with colleagues. This may be midwives who have recently undertaken evidence/research-based education activity, consultant midwives or midwifery lecturers. Often, the information generated through an evidence-based search is required by other midwives, so some local dissemination mechanism is a good idea. This may be through notice boards or meetings such as a journal club. The information may contribute to developing or updating clinical guidelines. Thus, this shortened EBP process has ongoing benefits in addition to answering a specific question. Figure 3.1 summarizes the shortened EBP process and the decision-making points in that process.

ACCESSING ORIGINAL LITERATURE/DATA: THE FULL EBP PROCESS

If you wish to access the original literature yourself, or have a question that has not been the subject of a systematic review, then a full evidence-based search is required. This does take more resources, and it may be appropriate that support is sought. Librarians are a very helpful resource. However, whether you seek support or not, you will need to access original data through a variety of search tools.

SEARCHING FOR THE ORIGINAL DATA

Probably the most well-known source is Medline. This is a huge database consisting of millions of entries on every subject related to healthcare. A good method of accessing Medline is via the National Library of Medicine (www.nlm.nih.gov). Remember to use American spellings as well as English ones, to think of alternative terms for the same thing, and to record each step you make so you can retrace your activities. Sackett et al. (2000) suggest that, despite the size of Medline, it still does not enable every paper on a topic to be identified; therefore, it is always worthwhile accessing profession-specific resources, for example MIDIRS and the RCM. Not only do these provide search facilities, but they also undertake searches for you for a stated cost. Other databases that may be of interest are the cumulative index for nursing and allied health literature (CINAHL), applied social sciences index and abstracts (ASSIA) and the web of science, which should be available through libraries. It is often useful to undertake a wider search of the internet using any of the search engines, as topic-specific websites including those for pregnant women often provide links to recent information. In addition, it is useful to scan profession-specific journals; again, their availability via the internet means that you can usually search for a topic over a number of volumes. Once you have identified a few possible articles, their reference lists may guide

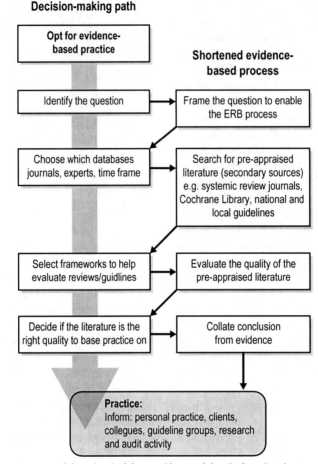

Figure 3.1 Flow diagram summarizing the decision making activity during the shortened evidence-based practice process.

you to other potential papers. Another good idea is to identify from the papers found any key researchers in the field and contact them directly.

The results of a detailed search should identify a series of papers, some of which will be research studies, while others may be reviews, audits, editorials and expert opinions. So, having identified the evidence the next stage is to access the papers. It may be possible to judge from abstracts whether or not a paper is relevant, but if in doubt it is always best to obtain the full report and to evaluate it. Sometimes topics have been studied more in one country than another, and although many authors (regardless of country of origin) do have their work published in English,

translation is rarely possible and this may restrict a complete review. On some topics this can mean obtaining a great number of articles/documents. Most libraries can get most publications, as can some organisations/professional bodies. If the evaluation is for a unit resource, such as a guideline, then deferring the costs to the organisation may be an option. Working in small groups is very useful, for peer support with the critical evaluation and to share the workload and expenses.

APPRAISING THE LITERATURE

Critical appraisal is the process by which the quality of an article/report is evaluated against set criteria, appropriate to the type of literature under scrutiny. It should look at every aspect of the paper and come to a balanced conclusion. The strengths and weakness of the processes involved should be assessed, along with the conclusions and implications for practice. To achieve this it is important to have a sound knowledge of the research process involved. This includes understanding the perspectives of the quantitative and qualitative paradigms, and the various approaches, designs, methods and tools that are used within research and most data collection activities. It is not possible to detail the full critical appraisal process here, but there are an increasing number of texts providing frameworks/guidance for the critical appraisal of evidence. This includes a variety of different types of evidence such as quantitative/qualitative research, audits, reviews, guidelines and expert opinion (Bluff and Cluett 2000, Crombie 1998, Greenhalgh 1997). The skills for critical appraisal include attention to detail, taking a logical approach and being prepared to read, and re-read, the evidence and then compare the evidence to information about what defines good practice in that particular research/data presentation format. A research textbook for reference is essential. Another useful exercise is to generate a table, identifying all the papers in the rows. In the columns identify the type of study, participants, inclusion criteria, who did the study, where and when, what the findings were, and the strengths and weaknesses. This gives a useful visual picture, and forms the basis of the decision-making processes of the appraisal. A collaborative approach can improve the quality of the conclusions by ensuring that nothing is overlooked and enhancing the analytical stages.

Although so far a broad definition of 'evidence' has been adopted, there is a hierarchy of evidence that informs decisions about the quality of any type of evidence. NICE (2003b) use the hierarchy presented in Table 3.1.

Aslam (2000) uses eight levels, which has RCTs as the highest level of evidence,

progressing down through non-experimental research, to personal experience, tradition and anecdotes. The limitation of both these hierarchies is the emphasis on quantitative data, and the exclusion of data from the qualitative paradigm. This may reflect the longer tradition of quantitative research within healthcare, its perceived objectivity and generalisability to populations, in comparison to qualitative research, which tends to be considered humanistic, and therefore subjective and context-related. Evidence-based practice as originally espoused was for individuals to receive the best care for them, and it is difficult to believe this can be achieved without consideration of qualitative literature. One possibility is to use qualitative sources to inform the way that the quantitative evidence is incorporated into practice. However, this could be considered to be relegating qualitative data to a lower level, which clearly is not the case, though this may be a starting point for the wider inclusion of qualitative research. Sackett et al. (2000), amongst others, have highlighted the dearth of qualitative research within systematic reviews, and acknowledge that nursing (and midwifery) are developing expertise in qualitative fields. Unfortunately, this has not yet translated into the incorporation

Table 3.1 Levels of Evidence

Level	Type of Evidence
1a	Meta-analysis of randomised controlled trials
1b	At least 1 randomised controlled trial
2a	At least 1 controlled study (no randomisation)
2b	At least 1 well-designed quasi-experimental study
3	Non-experimental descriptive studies, such as comparative studies, correlation, case-controlled studies
4	Expert committee reports or opinions and/or clinical experience of respected authorities

From: NICE 2003b Infection control: prevention of healthcare-associated infection in primary and community care. Clinical Guideline 2. NICE, London, p 23.
Adapted from White and Panjabi 1990.

of qualitative data/perspectives into the evidence-based literature.

At the end of the critical appraisal process several decisions are required. These include:

● which papers actually answer your question;
● which papers are of a good enough quality to consider the data they present;
● based on the best evidence what is/are the option(s) open to you and the client.

Figure 3.2 summarises the full EBP process and the decision-making points in that process. Having decided what is the best evidence, the next step is to put it into practice. While hopefully this is straightforward, the theory practice gap suggests that implementation is not easy.

Table 3.2 identifies the key stages of a short and full EBP search on water immersion during labour and birth, with some of the literature found.

IMPLEMENTATION OF THE EVIDENCE INTO PRACTICE

Implementing the evidence implies practising 'evidence-based practice' at all times. This should be the role of individual practitioners

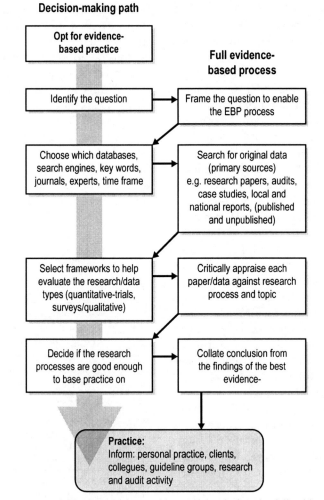

Figure 3.2 Flow diagram summarizing the decision making activity during the full evidence-based practice process.

Table 3.2   Stages and Results of Short and Full EBP Search Activity on Labour in Water

EBP Search Stage	Examples of Short Search Results	Examples of Full Search Results
Ask question	What is known about labour in water?	As short search
Frame question	Is labour in water safe? Does labouring in water reduce epidural analgesia use?	As short search
Search for pre-appraised literature	Cluett et al. (2004) in Cochrane Library. RCM (2000) position statement/guidelines	Not applicable
Search for original data	Not applicable	Trials identified in Cochrane review plus surveys by Alderdice et al. (1995), Gilbert and Tookey (1999), and comparative studies such as Richmond (2003)
Critically appraise literature	A review of RCTs only which suggests more research needed. Good practice guide only.	Small studies, limitation associated with inclusion criteria, care protocols and data collection.
Conclusion to take to practice	For women at low risk of complications reduces maternal reported pain experience and analgesia use, without apparently detrimental effects to woman and/or fetus/neonate. So, at the current time (and that's a caveat to all evidence), labour in water should be an option for women at low risk of complications.	

✎ Activity 3.2 Suggestion for Further Searches as a Learning Activity

Using Figures 3.1 and 3.2, and Table 3.2, try undertaking both a short and a full EBP search on the follow topics:

- One-to-one care during labour;
- Skin-to-skin contact to facilitate breast feeding;
- Nuchal fold translucency screening

Or any other topics that are pertinent to your practice.

This activity could be included in your portfolio as evidence of updating.

---

and everyone within units/services. This means making all clinically related decisions based on the best available evidence. It is important to consider the potential implications to practice that may occur. After collecting and critically appraising the evidence on a topic, and coming to conclusions for practice, several broad areas need to be considered. These include:

- Woman-centred factors
  - Is the evidence made available for women?
  - Is choice facilitated?
- Midwife factors
  - Are midwives educated/supported to provide this care?
- Service factors
  - Are there adequate resources in terms of equipment, suitable environment, numbers of trained midwives to provide appropriate care?
  - Are there guidelines for practice, interprofessional agreement where appropriate?
  - Are risk assessment/practice criteria agreed

Continuing the water immersion topic as an example, Box 3.3 highlights some of the questions that may need to be explored.

Box 3.3   Possible Issues Arising During the Decision-Making Process on Water Immersion During Labour and Birth

Possible initial questions

Do all the local units provide water birth facilities appropriate to local demand?

Is there information about the option and water birth workshops?

Can all or most midwives offer care to women in water?

Are there evidence-based and interprofessional local guidelines?

Are educational activities/support available for midwives developing skills in this area within the unit/trust?

Does the local educational institute include water immersion in their programmes?

The list can then be expanded to many other areas:

Does the local building have the environment/structures for a birth pool?

What is/would be the demand locally?

Are there enough midwives to offer this care, and provide the education, etc.?

If resources are put into pools, what are the consequences to other aspects of the budget?

Is having a pool cost-effective, or should resources be directed to socially deprived areas in order to make a difference and have a real impact on improving maternal and perinatal health?

Activity 3.3

Try identifying possible questions/resource implications for one of the evidence based searches conducted for the activity in Box 3.3

When just one relatively small topic is explored it becomes apparent why there is a gap between the evidence and the reality of practice, both in the United Kingdom and internationally (Villar et al. 2001, Richens 2002). The reasons for this are multiple and complex. It is too easy for midwives to blame management, and for management to blame funding. The barriers include all the things that affect any change process, fear of change, lack of knowledge, lack of support, organisational structures, and apathy, as well as time and resources. However, EBP will result in new practice implications being identified. The consequence of having decided to adopt EBP is that decisions will need to be made as to how to move forward to ensure that practice is evidence-based. To ensure that the evidence does influence practice is both a managerial and professional issue. Clinical governance activities should aid this, in particular the development of clear practice guidelines that are evidence-based. New ways of working with women, both within and across professions, provide the opportunities for EBP. The development of clinical leaders, such as consultant midwives, the evolving role of supervision of midwifery, education within the clinical setting as well as in universities including the availability of more postgraduate masters and doctorate-taught programmes, are all contributing to the change. Communication is much better nationally and internationally, with midwives sharing evidence and good practice. There are examples of excellence in practice now being shared via the internet (www.doh.gov.uk/deliveringthebest/index). All of these factors are contributing to a wider adoption of EBP, because it is the way to the provision of high-quality maternity care.

Women themselves are contributing to the development of evidence-based maternity services, by seeking out more information about the care options. Modern media and IT technology has fuelled this; many now have access to the internet, www.infochoice.org being an example of an information source for women and midwives. The work of consumer groups also has an important role in promoting EBP, and drawing attention to areas where evidence is neither implemented nor restricted. This should help ensure the widest understanding of EBP, with women's unique needs and preferences being part of the equation.

EVIDENCE-BASED PRACTICE AND CONFLICT

There are two potential areas of conflict, midwives and/or women-maternity service, and midwife-woman. Where the woman's wishes are supported by the evidence, but not within local guidelines/custom and practice, then the role of the midwife is to support the woman, be her advocate, and facilitate her care options. Start by ensuring that you have accessed the evidence and appraised it carefully, so you can provide the evidence at discussions with the supervisor of midwives, head of midwifery, and obstetrician. If any midwife does not feel empowered to do this, there should be a local support system of senior midwives, including consultant midwives and supervisors. Finding out the options available in other units may help. Contacting the RCM for information and/or support may be appropriate, as may be contacting a midwife with particular expertise in the topic. If the issue is totally within the sphere of midwifery practice, the provision of care in a midwifery-led unit, or in the woman's home may be an option. Through a combination of these approaches it should be possible to enable the woman to have the birth experience that is best for her. Indeed, it could be that this type of activity – though challenging for those involved at the time – has the potential to promote EBP in the unit, to generate guidelines, to update practitioners and to encourage interprofessional working. It almost makes it worth trying to find women to request the evidence you would like to see in practice; women and midwives working together for the health of all.

Negotiation is also the key to overcoming any potential difficulties where the woman's wishes are at odds with practice guidelines/ evidence. It is important to respect the wishes of the woman, and to ensure the decision she is making is fully informed and based on the best evidence. So the process is the same – access the literature, appraise it, and then provide that information to the woman in a usable, unbiased format and help her decide what is best for her (see Chapter 9 on helping women to make decisions). It may be that after this she makes a decision that reflects the best evidence, but the possibility remains that she does not, and her wishes must be respected. There are ethical dilemmas when there is debate as to the impact of the woman's choice to her fetus/neonate or her ability to make a choice is questioned. These dilemmas are outside the scope of this text, but are considered in Chapter 7.

EVALUATING EVIDENCE-BASED PRACTICE

Monitoring of the use of evidence and its impact on practice is being assessed. For example, Munro and Spilby (2003) report how the introduction of EBP guidelines has been shown to be influencing practice and the practice culture through an audit comparing practice before and after their introduction. Evaluative data needs to be collected locally and nationally, including birth outcomes such as operative deliveries, particularly as it has been suggested that EBP would reduce the Caesarean section rate in some places (Langer and Villar 2002). Other data that should be collected include hospitalisation, breast feeding, and the softer outcomes such as maternal satisfaction, midwifery retention as a marker of professional satisfaction with their role, to identify but a few possibilities. The cost-effective perspective could also be assessed, the initial cost of care, but also subsequent care needs or litigation. A national database of maternity statistics would provide the opportunity for comparison across units with or without the adoption of EBP. Auditing of practice on this level fits well with clinical governance and everyone's espoused agenda of improving the maternity service.

THE FUTURE: RESEARCH AND AUDIT FOR GENERATING THE EVIDENCE

If midwifery is to be a fully EBP profession, then there is a very urgent need for more high-quality evidence. This means maternity services, educational institutions, midwives and women undertaking, funding, supporting, and promoting research activity. One way of moving research forward in a coherent and meaningful way would be through national and local research agendas that explore the issues important to all the stakeholders. The auditing of practice, as suggested above, would not only monitor the effect of implementation of the evidence but also provide evidence for future practice. Thus, a reflective practice cycle is established, where practice is evaluated, evidence identified and appraised, decisions made on its value to practice and its implementation in practice, and the evidence is then implemented. This new practice is evaluated from the perspective of the women, the midwives and the service, and the cycle starts again.

SUMMARY AND CONCLUSIONS

Evidence-based practice is the linchpin to modern woman-centred maternity care. The first and most important decision for all in maternity services is to adopt the EBP philosophy and its processes. To enable this, all practitioners need education to understand the broad and full meaning of EBP. They need the time, resources and support to understand the process, including the decision making that is integral to the process. Evidence-based practice can only work if evidence is being updated and expanded, which implies that there is an ongoing need for research, audits and evaluation of practice. Consumers need to be involved in each step of these developments so that the emphasis remains on meeting the needs and preferences of women.

To achieve this, midwives will need to work in innovative ways to ensure that practice continues to develop. Methods of integrating qualitative data as well as quantitative data must be further explored, to ensure a humanistic approach and not merely a technocratic one. This implies not only educating current midwives, and all health practitioners, but also encouraging flexibility, creativity, and dynamic leadership within an open, learning, well-organised, managed and resourced environment. There are many forward-thinking individuals, groups, units working in just this manner and, like ripples in a pond, they will spread outwards.

KEY POINTS FOR BEST PRACTICE

- Evidence-based practice (EBP) is a philosophy and a practical way of working to ensure that clinical care is based on identifiable sources of evidence which are open for critical appraisal.

- EBP is the responsibility of individual midwives, but also managers, service providers and government – in fact, all who contribute to the maternity services.

- Evidence comes in many forms, including research and audit data, scientific and technological knowledge, personal and professional experience.

- The first and most important decision is to integrate EBP into everyday practice.

- The five-step EBP process: setting the question; collect the evidence; critique the evidence; apply the conclusions to practice; and evaluate the outcomes of the process– as well as practice-required decisions at every stage.

- Using pre-evaluated evidence in the form of national and local guidelines and systematic reviews is a valid and realistic option for most practitioners.

References

Albrecht G, Scholl WMJ, Basver A 2002 Mode of delivery and outcome of 699 term singleton breech deliveries at a single centre. American Journal of Obstetrics and Gynecology 87(6): 1694–1698.

Alderdice F, Renfrew M, Marchant S, Ashurst H, Hughes P, Berridge G, Garcia J 1995 Labour and birth in water in England and Wales. British Medical Journal 310: 837.

Aslam R 2000 Research and evidence in midwifery. In: Proctor S, Renfrew M (eds), Linking Research and Practice in Midwifery. A guide to evidence based practice. Baillière Tindall, Edinburgh, Chapter 1, pp. 15–34.

Bluff R, Cluett ER 2000 Critiquing the literature. In: Cluett ER, Bluff R (eds), Principles and Practice of Research In Midwifery. Baillière Tindall, Edinburgh, Chapter 10, pp. 179–196.

Cleverley D 2003 Implementing Inquiry Based Learning in Nursing. Routledge, London.

Cluett ER 2000 Experimental research. In: Cluett ER, Bluff R (eds), Principles and Practice of Research In Midwifery. Baillière Tindall, Edinburgh, Chapter 3, pp. 27–56.

Cluett ER, Nikodem C, McCandlish R, Burns E 2004 Immersion in water during pregnancy, labour and Childbirth. (Cochrane review). In: The Cochrane Library 2004. Issue 2 Update software, Oxford.

Crombie IK 1998 A pocket guide to critical appraisal. A handbook for health care professionals. BMJ Publishing group, London.

DaCruz D 2002 You Have a Choice, Dear Patient. British Medical Journal 324: 674.

Department of Health 1993 Changing Childbirth. Report of the expert maternity group. HMSO, London.

Department of Health 1997 The New NHS: Modern, Dependable. The Stationery Office, London.

Department of Health 1998 A First Class Service: quality in the NHS. HMSO, London.

Department of Health 1999 Clinical Governance: Quality in the New NHS. HMSO, London.

Evidence Based Practice Working Group 1992 Evidence based medicine: a new approach to teaching the practice of medicine. Journal of the American Medical Association 268: 2420–2425.

Gilbert RE, Tookey PA 1999 Perinatal mortality and morbidity among babies delivered in water; surveillance study and postal survey. British Medical Journal 319: 483–487.

Greenhalgh T 1997 How to read a paper? The basics of evidence based medicine. BMJ Publishing group, London.

Hannah M, Hannah W, Hewson S, Hodnett E, Saigal S, Willan A 2000 Planned caesarean section versus planned vaginal birth for breech presentation at term; a randomised multicentre trial. The Lancet 356(921): 1375–1383.

Haynes RB, Devereaux PJ, Guyatt GH 2002 Clinical expertise in the era of evidence-based medicine and patient choice [editorial]. ACP Journal Club; March-April 136: A11–A14.

Langer A, Villar J 2002 Promoting evidence based practice in maternal care would keep the knife away. British Medical Journal 324: 928–929.

Munro J, Spilby H 2003 Evidence into practice for midwifery led care: part 3. British Journal of Midwifery 11(7): 425–428.

National Institute for Clinical Excellence 2001 The use of electronic fetal monitoring. Clinical Guideline C. NICE, London.

National Institute for Clinical Excellence 2002 Guidance on the use of routine antenatal anti-D prophylaxis for RhD negative women. NICE, London.

National Institute for Clinical Excellence 2003a Antenatal care. Routine care for the healthy pregnant woman. Clinical Guideline 6. NICE, London.

National Institute for Clinical Excellence 2003b Infection control: prevention of healthcare-associated infection in primary and community care Clinical Guideline 2. NICE, London.

NHS Executive 1999 Clinical Governance: Quality in the new NHS. Department of Health, London.

NHS Executive 2000 The NHS plan. A plan for investment, a plan for reform. HMSO, London.

Price B 2003 Studying Nursing Using Problem Based and Enquiry Based Learning. Paulgrove. MacMillan, Basingstoke.

Proctor S, Renfrew M 2000 Introduction. In: Proctor S, Renfrew M (eds), Linking Research and Practice in Midwifery. A guide to evidence based practice. Baillière Tindall, Edinburgh, Chapter 1, pp. 1–11.

Richens Y 2002 Are midwives using research evidence in practice? British Journal of Midwifery 10(1): 11–16.

Richmond H 2003 Women's experience of waterbirth. Practising Midwife 6(3): 26–31.

Robinson J 2001 The breech birth trial – a consumer view. MIDIRS Midwifery Digest 11(3) Suppl. 2: S30–S32.

Rogers J 2002 Guidelines for intrapartum midwifery led care. International Confederation of Midwives. ICM proceeding CD-Rom. ICM, Vienna.

Royal College of Midwives 2000 The use of water in labour and birth. Position statement 1a. RCM London. (www.rcm.org.uk/info_centre/data/position_papers).

Royal College of Midwives 2002 Home birth. Position statement 25. RCM London. (www.rcm.org.uk/info_cemtre/data/position_papers).

Royal College of Obstetricians and Gynaecologists 2001 Clinical Green Top Guidelines: Thromboembolic Disease in Pregnancy and the Puerperium: Acute Management. Royal College of Obstetricians and Gynaecologists, London. (www.rcog.org.uk/guidelines).

Sackett DL, Rosenberg WMC, Gray JAM, Haynes RB, Richardson WS 1996 Evidence-based medicine: what it is and what it isn't. British Medical Journal 312: 71–72.

Sackett DL, Straus SE, Richardson WS, Rosenberg W, Haynes RB 2000 Evidence-based medicine: how to practice and teach EBM. 2nd edition. Churchill Livingstone, Edinburgh.

Villar J, Carroli G, Gulmezoglu M 2001 The gap between evidence and practice in maternal health care. International Journal of Obstetrics and Gynecology 75: S47–S54.

Further Reading

Buggins E, Nolan M 2000 Involving consumers in research. In: Proctor S, Renfrew M (eds), Linking Research and Practice in Midwifery. A guide to evidence based practice. Baillière Tindall, Edinburgh, Chapter 5, pp. 89–102.
This is a useful chapter in the context of woman-centred care.

Cluett ER, Bluff R (eds) 2000 Principles and Practice of Research in Midwifery. Baillière Tindall, Edinburgh.

This research text is recommended to readers to support the research related information presented in this chapter, especially Chapter 5 (pp. 79–112), which provides an introduction to understanding quantitative data/statistics in midwifery research.

Proctor S, Renfrew M (eds) 2000 Linking Research and Practice in Midwifery. A guide to evidence based practice. Baillière Tindall, Edinburgh.

A useful text to illustrate the interface between research and evidence-based care in midwifery practice.

Useful Websites

Please note that these sites are subject to change and relocation:
www.cebm.utoronto.ca/ebm: website supporting the Sackett et al. (2000) evidence-based medicine textbook
www.doh.gov.uk/deliveringthebest /index

www.infochoice.org
www.nlm.nih.gov
www.rcm.org.uk
www.rcog.org.uk
www.york.ac.uk/inst/crd

Chapter **4**

Models of Decision Making

Heidi Mok and Peggy A. Stevens

INTRODUCTION

According to Baumann and Deber (1989), decision making can be defined as the situation in which a choice is made among a number of possible alternatives, often involving a trade-off among the values given to different outcomes. This chapter will address various models of decision making. The intention is to present a set of principles that can help decisions to be made, rather than giving quick-fix answers to problems. Some examples will be used to uncover the processes involved. Readers are encouraged to work through the activities in order to enhance understanding of the individual models and its application to practice.

Decision making is a complex process in the everyday life of a midwife. Midwives must make decisions daily about whether a problem exists or has the potential for existing, what the cause of that problem is, and what intervention would be most beneficial for solving the problem (Ellis 1997). The use of the word 'problem' is, nonetheless, contentious within the context of midwifery, as childbearing and birth exist within a model of health rather than ill health. Even though traditionally the majority of midwives come from the nursing background, the concept of 'problem' has been widely contested as a way of embracing birth as a physiological event. Yet, in the light of increasing technological advances;

extending role of the traditional boundary of midwifery practice; quality-conscious culture; clinical negligence; clinical risk management; professional misconduct as portrayed in the Confidential Enquiries into Maternal Deaths (Lewis and Drife 2001) and Confidential Enquiry into Stillbirths and Deaths in Infancy report [CESDI] (Department of Health 2001) (as from April 2003, these two reports have been merged to form the Confidential Enquiry into Maternal and Child Health; see Lewis and Drife 2004), clinical decision-making skill is gaining momentum as an essential requisite for everyday midwifery practice.

Within the concept of accountability (as has been discussed in Chapters 1 and 7), the Nursing and Midwifery Council (NMC 2004) states that professionals are expected to make their own decision as part of that accountability. Midwives will be expected to base their decisions on evidence, and to be able to give their reasons when challenged. In order to reflect on their decision making, they must be aware of the processes and theories relating to decision making.

Adapted from Moody (1983), Box 4.1 highlights the essential ingredients in decision making.

Figure 4.1 demonstrates how the ingredients in Box 4.1 interrelate with the associating factors in midwifery clinical decision making.

The complexity of clinical decision making is a well-reported phenomenon. A review of the literature has shown that study in clinical decision making in midwifery is extremely limited, and has largely been informed by studies examining clinical decision making in medicine and in nursing. The earliest studies (Elstein and Bordage 1988) have demonstrated physicians and medical students using the hypothetico-deductive model based on the information processing theory to make diagnostic decisions. The seminal influential research of Newell and Simon (1972) established the basis of information processing theory, describing how the brain deals with the reception, storage and processing of information received from the environment.

Box 4.1 Ingredients in Decision Making

There are a number of ingredients in decision making:

- **Facts** - these can be described as concrete; black and white reality. They are transparent and can be taken from clients notes; laboratory reports; signs and symptoms and verbal history.
- **Knowledge** – this can be theoretical knowledge or of people or circumstances (Eraut 1994).
- **Experience** – this can be from the past or present and can be personal experience; the experience of others such as the mother, midwives and medical team.
- **Analysis** – this need to be undertaken before judgement(s) can be made. It could be objective as well as subjective. It forms the basis of the traditional approach to decision making.
- **Judgement** – this is a combination of all the above ingredients. It is similar to analysis that can be both objective and subjective. Judgment in midwifery practice needs to take account of clinical risk.

Source: Adapted from Moody P 1983 Decision Making. McGraw-Hill, New York.

HYPOTHETICO–DEDUCTIVE MODEL/SYSTEMATIC–POSITIVISTIC MODEL/RATIONALIST MODEL

The predominant approach to midwifery decision making until the 1980s has been the hypothetico-deductive rational process, derived from the field of cognitive psychology. It is depicted in the literature to be a rational and logical approach where an analysis of the situation could be made, and where knowledge and judgement could be made explicit. This means that the clinician, working with an unstructured problem, begins from a known starting point (main complaint) and proceeds along to an as-yet unknown end point.

The hypothetico-deductive model has been described in the following stages:

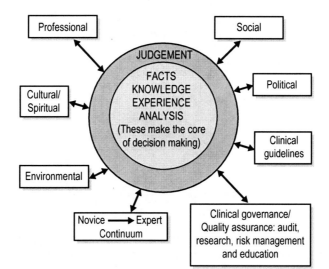

Figure 4.1   Midwifery clinical decision making.

- Select cues presenting in the situation;
- Generate hypothesis (typically stages 1–3, see Figure 4.2) relate to initial data and short-term memory;
- Selectively search for cues seeking confirmation or disconfirmation of hypotheses;
- Identify alternatives for action – weighing up pros and cons;
- Consider outcomes/risk attached/context.

Source: Adapted from Elstein A, Bordage G 1988 Psychology of Clinical Reasoning. In: Dowie J, Elstein A (eds), Professional Judgment: A Reader in Clinical Decision Making. Cambridge University Press, Cambridge, p. 112.

The example outlined in Figure 4.2 provides an explanation of how the stages in the hypothetico-deductive model can be interpreted.

Using the stages in the hypothetico-deductive model, the reader needs to work through Activity 4.1. The reader should consider the ingredients of decision making in order to make an informed judgement to generate a hypothesis.

Activity 4.1

A mother is complaining of feeling feverish and has extreme breast tenderness (unilateral) on day 7 in the post-natal period.

What could be the problem?

Although the hypothetico-deductive model is an efficient process, Harbison (2001) highlighted that it could be affected by a number of cognitive biases. One of these biases is 'anchoring', when the decision maker(s) tend to favour their initial hypothesis despite incoming contradictory evidence. In Figure 4.2, if the woman had a low platelet count the differential diagnosis could be bruising resulting from thrombocytopenia. In addition, hypothesis generation is often influenced by memory of similar cases, biased by previous experience.

The generation of the hypothesis in Figure 4.2 reduces the credibility of the final decision in the absence of testing, which is the key hallmark in the positivist approach. This leads to the use of the Bayesian approach (Hammond et al. 1967, Aspinall 1979) which enables the clinician to assess the probability of events, based on the logical interpretation of evidence. It is well accepted and established in fields outside midwifery. It enables people to deal with probabilities logically, in the sense that 2 + 2 equals 4.

BAYES' THEOREM – A RULE OF PROBABILITY

Bayes' theorem (which is also discussed in Chapter 5) argues that people hold degrees of belief in relation to scientific theories

The probability that a woman is a victim of domestic abuse will depend on:
- How sensitive an indicator the diagnostic evidence is (eg. the amount of bruising, non-verbal communication)
- How far the diagnostic evidence can be confined to abuse victims
- How prevalent is abuse in the population
- Your experience in dealing with victims of abuse
  See below for hypothesis testing

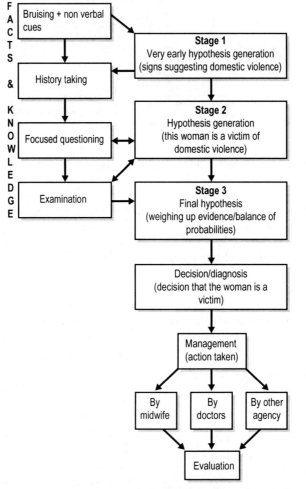

Figure 4.2   An example of how the stages in the hypothetico-deductive model can be interpreted.

(or indeed any phenomenon). Moreover, these degrees of belief will be adjusted in response to the presentation of new probability or evidence (Thompson 1999). Hammond et al. (1967) examined the ways in which six nurses revised their diagnosis of patients' conditions as new data were gathered and presented. These revised hypotheses were then compared with calculated probabilities of the conditions.

Whilst consistently reviewing their hypothesis, the nurses tended to be 'cognitively cautious' in their revisions. This relates to what Harbison (2001) calls 'anchoring'.

Doubilet and McNeil (1988) took this approach further and developed a 'decision tree' which is used to display the possible decision options of the problem under consideration. The tree gives the possible consequences of each option. Probabilities (likelihood that the outcome will occur) are attached to these alongside subjective utilities, or values placed on each possible outcome.

Objective determination of probabilities derives from knowledge of the data about an appropriate group of clients in which the final outcome and state of each is recorded. However, some would argue that risk is socially constructed and never objective, even when probabilities are derived. Subjective probability on the other hand, is based on the expert's own estimates. Along with probabilities, 'utility' or 'values' are assigned to each of the outcomes. This value should, where possible, be the client's expressed value. By multiplying the probability of each outcome with the assigned value, the expected value of each of the outcomes can be computed. The outcome with the highest expected value is regarded as the optimal choice.

Putting the above in the context of midwifery practice, the example depicted in Table 4.1 considers the decision regarding the options of rupturing or not rupturing the membranes. The factors to be taken into consideration are maternal and fetal safety and the length of

labour. The list could be extended depending on circumstances.

The probability of outcome is based on the midwife's understanding of the ingredients of decision making (facts, knowledge, experience, analysis and judgement) together with subjective estimates of possible outcome. Therefore, all of the stated probabilities will be unique to the individual midwife.

The utility value is based on the woman's understanding of her needs. The value is normally measured as a percentage and is thus between 0 and 100. As the woman has requested the membranes to be left intact, her value will be low under the option of artificial rupture of membranes. However, she may be persuaded that in the light of fetal compromise an artificial rupture of membranes will be beneficial and consent given to undertake the procedure; thus a score of 70. As the woman requested a natural birth, the value placed on the speeding up of labour is of low value; thus a value of 0.

For the 'no artificial rupture of membranes' option exactly the same factors of maternal and fetal safety and length of labour need to be considered. The probability of outcome for

---

Table 4.1 Example Decision Tree. A primigravid woman is in labour with a cervical dilatation of 4 cm. The midwife is considering if she should leave the membranes intact as the woman has requested for 'natural' birth. The unit policy implies that membranes should be ruptured

			Probability of Outcome (Midwife)		Utility (Value) (Mother)		Expected Value	Overall Value
		Maternal safety	0.9	×	0	=	0	
	A.R.M.	Fetal safety	0.7	×	70	=	49	49
		Length of labour	0.9	×	0	=	0	
Options		Maternal safety	1	×	100	=	100	
	No A.R.M.	Fetal safety	0.2	×	80	=	16	126
		Length of labour	0.1	×	100	=	10	
			Scale 0–1		Scale 0–100			
			(0 = not possible)		(high score = high value)			
			(1 = certainty)					

Source: Adapted from Doubilet P, McNeil B 1988 Clinical Decision Making. In: Dowie J, Elstein A (eds), Professional Judgment: A Reader in Clinical Decision Making. Cambridge University Press, Cambridge, p. 257.

maternal safety related to the 'no intervention'. The 0.2 probability takes account of the potential risk of existence of meconium-stained liquor. The 0.1 probability for the length of labour relates to the empirical evidence that labour can be shortened by approximately 1 hour following artificial rupture of membranes.

The expected value is derived from multiplying the probability and utility values for each factor. The overall value is the sum of all expected values in each option. In the light of overall value of 49 for the artificial rupture of membranes option and 126 for the no artificial rupture of membranes option which gives a 126:49 ratio, the midwife can be justified to leave the membranes intact.

This is a technique specifically designed for unique decisions that are complex, where there may be uncertainty, and which are value-laden, as shown by the example above. This is particularly pertinent in today's society when women are better informed and more prepared to ask questions and to expect a partnership in maternity care. This model will form the basis to an informed debate based on the midwife's clinical experience and the woman's personal situation.

By utilizing such a process, expert practitioners would be able to assist novices to develop their decision-making skills. Owing to its mathematical orientation, the use of this model may be limited; however, this approach enables the midwife to rationalize the tacit (taken-for-granted) element in their decision making.

✎ Activity 4.2

Using the decision tree in Table 4.1, work out the options, probabilities, utility values, expected values, and overall values in order to justify your decision when undertaking the following activity:

A multigravida is in her late pregnancy. She says that she intends to place her baby on its tummy to settle. She did this with the previous two children without problems and they did not succumb to Sudden Infant Death Syndrome.

What is your response?

DIFFERENTIATIONS FROM OTHER APPROACHES

It is clear that the systematic positivist approach is prescriptive rather than descriptive. This has the potential to improve decision making, particularly for the novice midwife due to its logical, sequential process. However, it does not take full account of the reality of clinical practice. In practice, midwives frequently overlap stages in the decision-making process and change their order, thus forming the basis for the competing, intuitive-humanistic model of clinical decision making.

THE INTUITIVE–HUMANISTIC MODEL/PHENOMENOLOGICAL PERSPECTIVE

The main principle behind all intuitive–humanist models (which is also explored in Chapter 2) is that intuitive judgement distinguishes the expert from the novice, with the expert no longer relying on analytical principles to connect their understanding of the situation to appropriate action.

Those who hold this view contend that there are limits to the use of traditional or rational strategies of decision making as experienced midwives see and use patterns in the whole situation rather than reducing the situation to discrete parts. In the process of analysing the parts, sensitivity could be lost and the basis for decision making is weakened. This perspective accords with the holistic view of midwifery care.

Intuition, or 'gut feeling', has seldom been granted legitimacy as a sound approach as it is not congruent with the philosophy of logical positivism. However, much of the literature on decision making includes intuition as part of the process of decision making (Benner 1984, Orme and Maggs 1993). Overall, intuition allows the midwife to arrive at a rapid (often subliminal) judgement based on visual, verbal and non-verbal cues, or to detect missing data or gaps in the information, or enables the possibility of gaining information directly about the future. Returning to the example in Table 4.1, the physical signs and the midwife's intuitive knowledge would lead her to seek out the missing data to confirm the possible judgement of domestic violence or other differential causes.

Pattern recognition is another type of heuristics used by midwives in interpreting data for problem solving. Pattern recognition or 'representativeness' is the process of making a judgement on the basis of a few critical pieces of information. This means that expert reasoning in non-problematic situations closely resembles pattern matching or direct automatic retrieval from well-structured networks of stored knowledge (Offredy 1998). Thus, a new case is categorized by its similarity to a client seen earlier and is, therefore, given the same diagnosis. In the example in Table 4.1, domestic violence could be made on the basis of an earlier experience (personal or professional). This is in accord with research undertaken by Cioffi and Markham (1997) into clinical decision making, that clinicians based their decision upon representativeness (how it relates to previous experience); availability (how easy it is to recall); and anchoring adjustment (favouring originally held beliefs, but some adjustment on the basis of new evidence). The difference between the novice and the expert can be explained in terms of the size of the knowledge store of previous experience(s) available for pattern recognition.

Many midwives will acknowledge the role that intuition or 'gut feelings' play in their practice. Benner (1984) contends that the use of intuition is a legitimate part of midwifery practice, and has described aspects of intuitive judgment such as:

* pattern and similarity recognition
* common sense understanding (derived from knowledge of culture, society and language)
* skilled 'know-how'
* sense of salience (distinguishing meaningful events)
* deliberative rationality (adopting a new perspective on a situation).

The main difference between pattern recognition and intuition is that intuition occurs at an unconscious level, whereas pattern recognition occurs at a conscious level (Benner 1984).

The example in Box 4.2 demonstrates the difference between pattern recognition and intuition.

The 'messiness' of reality in practice means that midwives need to develop the skills to cope with the uniqueness, uncertainty and conflict inherent in each situation. It would be extremely simplistic to adopt one perspective to the exclusion of the other. As a result, most midwives use an eclectic approach to decision

---

Box 4.2

A woman at 32 weeks' gestation is complaining of 'feeling puffy', and in particular in her extremities.

* What are the probable signs and symptoms of pre-eclampsia ?
* The majority of women have oedema of some sort during pregnancy.
* Careful questioning has shown that the woman is struggling between a busy home and work life, and is planning to work into late pregnancy.
* Are there other discernable signs that may alert you to the potential risks?
* Has there been previous history (medical, obstetric or familial) which might have increased the risks?
* What is your 'gut feeling' telling you?

The midwife would consciously recollect the signs and symptoms of pre-eclampsia as well as previous cases attended (pattern recognition). This would lead the midwife to investigate pertinent questions which may confirm or dispel the original hypothesis of pre-eclampsia. In the absence of positive signs and symptoms, the midwife would still trust her intuitive judgment (intuition) that a woman 'feeling puffy' is not normal. This would lead her to decide that this woman will require closer monitoring in the absence of a firm diagnosis.

making. One of these examples could be demonstrated by Orme and Maggs' (1993) stages of decision making below.

In their study on how expert nurses, midwives and health visitors make clinical decisions, Orme and Maggs (1993) found that decision making must be based on a sound knowledge base, may involve risk taking, and must take place within a supportive environment with a shared philosophy of care. However, all decisions must be taken with the safety of the client as paramount. Orme and Maggs' (1993) study identified a number of stages in the decision-making process (see Table 4.2).

In order for the reader to become conversant with Orme and Maggs' (1993) stages of decision making, it is suggested that Activity 4.3 is undertaken using the model provided in Table 4.2.

✎ Activity 4.3

Explore how the midwife would discuss the option of water-birth.

As previously identified in this chapter, decision-making is part of the midwife's everyday practice. Cole (1996) considers decision making in managerial role stating that decisions are made ". . . on the spur of the moment; or after much thought and deliberation; or somewhere between the two extremes". Cole's (1996) theories on decision making have relevance to midwifery practice, because midwives make on-the-spur-of-the-moment decisions; or after much thought and consideration decisions; or decisions somewhere along this continuum in everyday midwifery practice. Cole's (1996) principles and how they can be related to midwifery practice and the traditional approach to decision making will now be explored.

SPUR-OF-THE-MOMENT DECISIONS IN RELATION TO MIDWIFERY PRACTICE

The decisions made about the management of maternity/neonatal emergencies such as eclampsia or neonatal asphyxia could be considered as spur-of-the-moment decisions, as

Table 4.2   Stages in Decision Making

Stage 1	Establish a philosophy of care which provides the framework within which decisions can be made.
Stage 2	Determine whether the decision is necessary and can you (as opposed to someone else) make it?
Stage 3	Assess the whole situation.
Stage 4	Explore and examine all possible courses of action, including client and practitioner intuitive feelings; ethical, legal and moral issues; available resources; knowledge and research findings; conflicts of interest; code of professional conduct; views of nursing and multidisciplinary teams; and past experience of similar situations.
Stage 5	Select course of actions and inform 'concerned others' of the rationale behind the decision.
Stage 6	Implement action and monitor implementation.
Stage 7	Reflect on both the outcome and the decision-making process.

Reproduced with permission from: Orme L, Maggs C 1993 Decision making in clinical practice: how do expert nurses, midwives and health visitors make decisions? Nurse Education Today 13: 270–276. © Harcourt Publishers Ltd.

any delay in management could be detrimental for either mother or baby, or both. Put in the context of maternity and neonatal emergencies, spur-of-the-moment decisions are therefore an inevitable part of midwifery practice. However, it is important to emphasise that this does not imply that no thought and consideration goes into the management of such situations, because as humans we think about and consider any situation we encounter. Spur-of-the-moment decisions for maternity and neonatal emergencies however are usually based on written guidelines where specific steps are followed, for example ABC for resuscitation.

Most of the thought and consideration process which follows the principles of the traditional decision-making process has taken place during the process of producing such guidelines for midwifery practice. The step-by-step guidelines for emergency situations are concomitant with the linear progression of the traditional approach to decision making, as described previously in the hypothetico-deductive model. The formulation of the guidelines are not based on emotions, feelings or interpersonal relations, but are 'rational' (Cole 1996), in that they are based on deductive reasoning. They move from identifying the problem to selecting and implementing the appropriate course of action and then measuring results in terms of success of the management. Similarities to this process can be seen in the quantitative approach to research, which has a hypothetico-deduction process. Within both of these processes there is no room for subjectivity. The evidence or guidelines are based on objectivity and not subjectivity.

It could also be argued that for spur-of-the-moment decisions in maternity emergencies a substantial amount of thought and consideration process also takes place after the event, when the midwife reflects on the care of the woman and/or baby. Thus, the midwife is engaging in what Schon (1987) calls reflection on action (also addressed in Chapter 10). This process demonstrates how the midwife has moved along the decision-making continuum.

Whilst it is interesting to apply spur-of-the-moment decisions to maternity emergencies, many may perceive such decisions as being based on some irrational process that has no real structure or order. Disorderly decision making does not conform to a traditional approach. Models such as the hypothetico-deductive, systematic-positivistic and rationalist models are entrenched in rational and logical analysis of the situation where knowledge and judgement are made explicit.

THOUGHT AND CONSIDERATION AS PART OF DECISION MAKING IN MIDWIFERY PRACTICE

Cole (1996) describes the other end of the decision-making continuum as being involved in much thought and consideration before decisions are reached. The management of a woman with social problems may be decided after much thought and consideration, as decisions are made after dialogue with the woman and member of the multi-professional team.

Although a decision has to be reached the urgency to initiate care is not the same as in a maternity/neonatal emergency. Such an approach to decision making again fits well into traditional/rational models. As previously discussed, all models require a logical, sequential and analytical approach where the situation is analysed and possible solutions are considered and rejected before an optimum solution is reached. Whilst this is a rational, logical, sequential and analytical process, it could be argued that due to the lack of urgency there is time to consider emotions, feelings and interpersonal relationships in the decision-making process when the situation is explored and alternative and final solutions are reached. This demonstrates how a range of decision-making models can be used to arrive at an appropriate decision.

THE CONTINUUM OF DECISION MAKING

It could be argued however that most of the decisions made by midwives in their everyday practice are along a continuum of these two extremes. For example, the management of a post-natal woman who is having problems with breast feeding is both immediate and ongoing. Decision about care may be needed quickly (spur-of-the-moment), but thought and consideration are also needed when making them because step-to-step guidelines may not exist for such situations. Ongoing care decisions should be based on thought and consideration to achieve the quality of care advocated by Changing Childbirth (DoH 1993). Quality can be achieved through a combination of decision-making models. The choice of model will be dependent on the clinical situation and the midwife's experience.

The following 'middle ground' approach, as suggested by Thompson (1999), could be used to reconcile the opposing extremes of thinking. This 'middle ground' can be represented by Hamm's (1988) cognitive continuum theory which serves to represent the reality of practice (see Figure 4.3).

This theory indicates that for ill-structured tasks, with a large number of cues and very

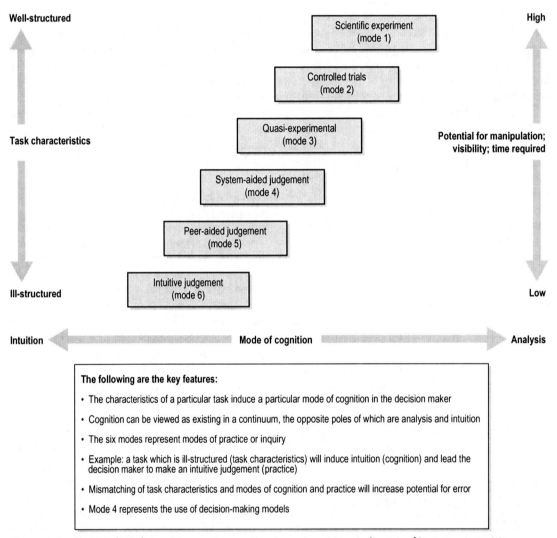

Figure 4.3   Hamm's (1988) cognitive continuum: the six modes of enquiry/practice [Source: adapted from Hamm RM 1988 Clinical intuition and clinical analysis: expertise and the cognitive continuum. In: Dowie J, Elstein A (eds), Professional Judgment: A Reader in Clinical Decision Making. Cambridge University Press, Cambridge, p. 87].

little time, intuition is the most appropriate cognitive mode to use. In well-structured tasks, with few cues and a lot of time, then analysis is the favoured cognitive mode. However, most tasks are a mixture of ill- and well-structured, and therefore fall somewhere in the middle of the continuum.

Hamm's (1988) and Cole's (1996) theoretical models/principles demonstrate two opinions on the continuum of decision making. Some may argue that they are similar as they both imply the movement of decision making along the continuum. However, as previously suggested, there is a discernible difference between the two perspectives in that a 'spur-of-the-moment' decision is not necessarily ill-structured.

Box 4.3 provides an example of how Hamm's (1988) model can be interpreted in midwifery practice.

ASSESSMENT OF RISK

Regardless of the model of decision making used, the individual midwife's judgement should not be reached without due consideration of the risks involved. The traditional or rational approach, and in particular the use of the Doubilet and McNeil (1988) decision tree, enables the midwife to compile the risk-benefit ratio. For all midwives – but in particular the novice midwife – the traditional or rational approach provide a framework in which to critically analyse situation, develop a hypothesis and risk ratio using the ingredients of facts, knowledge, experience and analysis to reach the optimal judgement of the situation.

CONCLUSION

Clinical decision making is a highly complex phenomenon. This is evident from the literature in this field of study. There is no one accepted theoretical or evidence-based model of clinical decision making. Indeed, the purpose of detailing the various models of decision making is not to seek a descriptive fit on what midwives actually do. This chapter on the traditional or rational approaches to clinical decision making should enable the readers to construct their own personal interpretation of clinical reasoning from the spectrum of ideas and perspectives that is presented. By being more explicit about the types of decision required of midwives, it is possible to establish what quality care is in midwifery practice.

According to Paul (1993), critical thinking is the art of thinking about your thinking while you are thinking to make your thinking better; more clear; more accurate, or more defensible. Models of decision making through a structured process should enable midwives and

Box 4.3

Jane has had a Caesarean section performed under epidural anaesthesia. Twelve hours later, she is accompanied to the bathroom by the midwife. She subsequently looks pale, complains of feeling faint and shows signs of central cyanosis. Help is summoned. A few seconds later, Jane experiences a convulsive seizure.

Using Hamm's (1988) cognitive continuum theory and following the key features, the midwife recognised the potential seriousness of Jane's condition prior to the convulsions. This led her to summon help even though a definite diagnosis had not been made (*mode 6* intuitive judgement). As soon as help arrived, a peer–aided judgement (*mode 5*) was able to be made. If there was a mismatch of understanding of the situation, errors in clinical decision and management can be made. To move to *mode 4*, policy and unit guidelines should come into place to enable appropriate action to be taken, e.g. caring during seizure.

There is a possibility of moving on along the continuum if the midwife is fully conversant with enquiry-based practice. Thus, she is able to recall and utilise the findings of relevant evidence. It is more likely that *modes 1* to *3* will take place after the event while reflecting on action.

student midwives to enhance their critical thinking abilities. After all, effective midwifery practice is about thinking and doing.

KEY POINTS FOR BEST PRACTICE

- Decision making is an inherent part of the midwife's professional life and should be based on up-to-date evidence.

- If based on evidence, all decisions should be open to challenge.

- It is essential that the midwife reflects on their decision making.

- To be able to make decisions, the midwife must be aware of the theories relating to decision making.

- Decision making is a complex process that includes a number of ingredients.

These are: facts; knowledge; experience; analysis; and judgement.

- The predominant approach to midwifery decision making until the 1980s was the rational and logical, hypothetical deductive model. Some midwives may still use this model.

- The model of decision making that a midwife utilises will be dependent on her/his clinical experience. Novices tend to utilise a more traditional model of decision making, whilst experts are able to apply intuition or 'gut feeling'.

- Midwives usually adopt more than one perspective to decision making, and this will be dependent on whether the decision is spur of the moment as in an emergency or after much thought and consideration.

References

Aspinall M 1979 Use of a decision tree to improve accuracy of diagnosis. Nursing Research 28: 182–185.

Baumann A, Deber R 1989 Limits of decision analysis for rapid decision making in ICU nursing. Image: Journal of Nursing Scholarship 21: 69–71.

Benner P 1984 From Novice to Expert. Addison Wesley, London.

Cioffi J, Markham R 1997 Clinical decision making by midwives: managing case complexity. Journal of Advanced Nursing 25: 265–272.

Cole GA 1996 Management Theory and Practice, 5th edition. Letts Educational, London.

Department of Health 1993 Changing Childbirth: Report of the expert maternity group. HMSO, London.

Department of Health 2001 Confidential Enquiry into Stillbirths and Deaths in Infancy. 8th Annual Report. Maternal and Child Health Research Consortium, London.

Doubilet P, McNeil B 1988 Clinical Decision making. In: Dowie J, Elstein A (eds), Professional Judgment: A Reader in Clinical Decision Making. Cambridge University Press, Cambridge.

Ellis P 1997 Processes used by nurses to make decisions in the clinical practice settings. Nurse Education Today 17: 325–332

Elstein A, Bordage G 1988 Psychology of clinical reasoning. In: Dowie J, Elstein A (eds), Professional Judgment: A Reader in Clinical Decision Making. Cambridge University Press, Cambridge.

Eraut M 1994 Developing Professional Knowledge and Competence. Falmer Press, London.

Hamm RM 1988 Clinical intuition and clinical analysis: expertise and the cognitive continuum. In: Dowie J, Elstein A (eds), Professional Judgment: A Reader in Clinical Decision Making. Cambridge University Press, Cambridge.

Hammond K, Kelly K, Scheider R, Vancini M 1967 Clinical inference in nursing: revising judgments. Nursing Research 16: 38–45.

Harbison J 2001 Clinical decision making in nursing: theoretical perspectives and their relevance to practice. Journal of Advanced Nursing 35(1): 126–133.

Lewis G, Drife J (eds) 2001 Why Mothers Die 1997–1999: The Confidential Enquiries into Maternal Deaths in the United Kingdom. The Fifth Report. RCOG, London.

Lewis G, Drife J (eds) 2004 Confidential Enquiry into Maternal and Child Health; Why Mothers Die 2000–2002. Sixth Report of the Confidential Enquiries into Maternal Deaths in the UK. RCOG Press, London.

Moody P 1983 Decision Making. McGraw-Hill, New York.

Newell A, Simon HA 1972 Human Problem Solving. Prentice-Hall, New Jersey.

Nursing and Midwifery Council 2004 Code of Professional Conduct: standards for conduct, performance and ethics. NMC, London.

Offredy M 1998 The application of decision making concepts by nurse practitioners in general practice. Journal of Advanced Nursing 28(5): 988–1000.

Orme L, Maggs C 1993 Decision making in clinical practice: how do expert nurses, midwives and health visitors make decisions? Nurse Education Today 13: 270–276.

Paul R 1993 Critical thinking: what every person needs to survive in a rapidly changing world. Centre for Critical Thinking, California.

Schon D 1987 Educating the Reflective Practitioner. San Francisco: Jossey-Bass

Thompson C 1999 A conceptual treadmill: the need for middle ground in clinical decision making theory in nursing. Journal of Advanced Nursing 30(5): 1222–1229.

Further Reading

Boney J, Baker JD 1997 Strategies for teaching clinical decision-making. Nurse Education Today 17: 16–21.

Bucknall T, Thomas S 1997 Nurses' reflections on problems associated with decision-making in critical care settings. Journal of Advanced Nursing 25: 229–237.

Claxton K, Sculpher M, Drummond M 2002 A rational framework for decision making by the National Institute for Clinical Excellence (NICE). Lancet 360(9334): 711–715.

Edwards N 2003 The choice is yours – or is it? AIMS Journal 15(3): 9–12.

English I 1993 Intuition as a function of the expert nurse: a critique of Benner's novice to expert model. Journal of Advanced Nursing 18: 387–393.

Hadikin R 2002 How fear drives your decision making. Practising Midwife 5(6): 36.

Jenks J 1993 The pattern of personal knowing in nurse clinical decision making. Journal of Nursing Education 32(9): 399–405.

Porzsott F, Ohletz A, Thim A, et al. 2003 Evidence-based decision making – the six step approach. Evidence Based Medicine 8(6): 165–166.

Thomson A 2003 Where has evidence come from, what do we have now and what will we have in the future. Midwifery 19: 1–2.

Watson S 1994 An exploratory study into a methodology for the examination of decision making by nurses in the clinical area. Journal of Advanced Nursing 20: 351–360.

Chapter **5**

Processes and Challenges in Clinical Decision Making

Marianne Mead and Amanda Sullivan

INTRODUCTION

Previous chapters have looked at the quality of knowledge and how knowledge can be used to support decision making and evidence-based practice. It may seem that, if midwives were able to retrieve and critique research, decision making would be easy. However, even simple decisions are quite complex and involve many factors. This chapter will explore some of the challenges involved. In particular, it will consider difficulties when interpreting clinical information to inform practice. The use of decision analysis will also be discussed. This is a way of identifying explicitly all choices and outcomes, assigning values to each outcome, and then reaching the optimal decision.

The art of medicine – and by extension, the art of midwifery – is the skilled application of medical science (Haynes de Regt et al. 1986), the processing of information (Barrett et al. 1990), or the choice of decision (Thornton 1990). Midwifery, like medicine, is not an exact science and errors are common. For decades, the confidential enquiries into maternal deaths (Lewis and Drife 2001) and, more recently, its child counterpart (Confidential Enquiry into Stillbirths and Deaths in Infancy 2001), have identified important areas of error or sub-standard decisions that have contributed to maternal or neonatal fatalities. (See also Lewis and Drife 2004.)

The processes used in medical diagnosis and treatment decisions have been subjected to a large amount of research (Bell et al. 1988; de Tombal 1988; Eraker and Politser 1982; Haynes de Regt et al. 1986; Johnson 1955; Kahneman et al. 1982; Kozielecki 1981; Tversky and Kahneman 1974). There is now much greater emphasis on the examination of the extent and potential causes of medical errors or near misses (Elstein et al. 1978; Weed and Weed 1999; Weingart et al. 2000).

ERRORS – WE ALL MAKE MISTAKES!

A divorce rate of about 50% and the high proportion of unplanned pregnancies suggest that people make a lot of mistakes. If errors are common in important personal issues, they are likely to be even more common in less personal areas, such as professional issues. So why is this? Box 5.1 presents a relatively common scenario that demonstrates how an initial error of diagnosis inevitably led to the wrong treatment advice.

Errors can be made at the point of diagnosis, or at the point of treatment options. In this context, judgement deals mainly with the correct evaluation of the information provided to decide whether a condition is present or not, and decision analysis deals with the weighting of options that will lead to optimum choices of treatments or interventions (McCaughan 2002).

THE NATURE OF DECISION ERRORS

Problems in human decision making may be related to the inability of human beings to process large amounts of information at the same time. This leads individuals to over-simplification and errors. But there is also evidence that increased information, and even understanding of that information, can fail to alter behaviour (Hamm 2000).

Medical students and physicians have been the main subjects of research on clinical diagnosis and error, but the principles apply to midwives and other healthcare professionals.

Box 5.1 Judgement and Decision

Yesterday, James fell while ice-skating. He tried to protect himself and in the process injured his wrist. This quickly became very swollen. He attended the local casualty department. An X-ray was taken and read, and he was reassured that nothing was broken. A small compression bandage was applied and he was discharged home.
JUDGEMENT – NO FRACTURE

The following evening, James received a phone call from the casualty department. A more experienced radiologist had reviewed his X-ray and had detected a fracture. James was advised to attend the fracture clinic for further treatment.
ERROR – DIAGNOSIS OF NO FRACTURE WHEN FRACTURE PRESENT

James attended the fracture clinic and a plaster cast was applied. James was now complaining of some significant pain. At this point, weighing carefully the advantages and disadvantages of various drugs, James was issued with a prescription for analgesics
DECISION ANALYSIS – TREATMENT

It is worth remembering that all the practitioners concerned were practitioners who did the best they could. Nevertheless, an error occurred.

Clinicians frequently question the processes they should use to arrive at a diagnosis. This is one of the most important and intellectually challenging aspects of medical reasoning (DeGowin and DeGowin 1969). Training which includes tutoring with more senior staff can result in newer staff accepting the methods of reasoning adopted by those they see as clinical experts (Bursztajn et al. 1988). Anecdotal evidence suggests that student midwives and midwives behave in the same way, and research supports the idea that the influence exercised by senior or influential members of staff is very important (Kirkham 1999).

THOUGHT PROCESSES AND DECISION-MAKING ERRORS

Arriving at a diagnosis involves thought processes, and medical textbooks are full of 'how' and 'what' to do, but decision makers are frequently unable to articulate their decision processes or the weight they allocate to individual sign or symptom (Kirwan et al. 1983). The approach is often intuitive. In this context, intuition can be defined as ". . .the ability to reach sound conclusions with minimal evidence. . ." (Wescott 1968), as ". . . understanding without rationale..." (Benner 1984), or ". . .immediate knowing of something without the conscious use of reason. . ." (Schrader and Fischer 1987). This has been illustrated by the examples of the expert professor reaching a diagnosis or treatment decision on the basis of apparently systematic consideration of the evidence presented by the patient, and the simultaneous reference to informal rules of thumb that cannot be reasoned (Bursztajn et al. 1988). For some, intuition has indeed been seen as the mark of the good clinician (Berlin and Marsh 1993), whereas others still explain this apparent lack of systematic analysis of a problem as the result of experience and knowledge stored in the 'background' (Sackett et al. 2000).

The combination of both logical problem-solving approaches and intuitive creative approaches has been seen as useful in enabling individuals to deal with facts and feelings and to make faster and more accurate decisions (Benner and Tanner 1987, Snyder 1993). Indeed, it has been suggested that expert nurses are able, through experience and critical thinking, to integrate analytic and logical problem-solving (Benner 1984). But intuition has been criticised as less analytic and structured than decisions made on the basis of peer-aided judgement, system-aided judgement, quasi-experimental studies, controlled trials and scientific experiment.

The outcome of many clinical situations involves some degree of uncertainty. Uncertainty can creep in at all levels of clinical practice, from defining a disease to making a diagnosis. It is important to appreciate how complex these tasks are, how poorly they are understood, and how easy it is for individuals to come to different conclusions when presented with the same information (Eddy 1984). The tendency to over-simplify complex information means that a high cure rate may be associated with an absolute cure rate in the mind of clinicians (Peschel and Peschel 1990). Likewise, a 'normal' or 'low-risk' pregnancy may be associated with the perception of an absolute chance of a positive outcome for parents and professionals alike. This can add to the distress of adverse outcomes.

"The evidence of the study of medical practitioners indicates that their attitude to uncertainty is ambivalent – aware of it when discussing its theoretical aspects but oblivious when preoccupied with its practical concerns" (Katz 1988). The explanations for not making parents aware of uncertainties can be based on either a perception of the inability of parents to make sense of the alternatives, or a concern for increasing their worry. The problem may therefore not only be one of the uncertainty itself but of the ability to remain mindful of, and indeed willing to acknowledge, uncertainty.

OTHER INFLUENCING FACTORS

The rates of accurate and erroneous diagnoses suggest that different factors ought to be taken in consideration when considering their potential accuracy. These involve the incidence or prevalence of a condition, the sensitivity and specificity of a test, and the effects of a positive or negative diagnosis.

Incidence is the number of new cases that occur during a specified period in a defined population. The prevalence of a condition is the number of people with the condition in a particular population at a point in time (Farmer et al. 1996). Clinicians are more likely to think of common problems when making a diagnosis. For example, breast lumps during pregnancy and lactation are more commonly associated with hormonal changes than malignancy. Midwives encountering this are more likely to consider hormonal changes than malignancy. As such, rare problems are more likely to be missed.

Decisions are also influenced by clinical signs and test results. However, some tests are more reliable than others. Two concepts are at play here – the actual presence or absence of a condition or disease and the positive or negative test results. These are not the same thing as Box 5.2 demonstrates.

The **sensitivity** or **true positive rate (TP)** of a test refers to the ability of the test to identify correctly the people who have a condition. **Specificity** or true negative rate (TN) refers to the ability of the test to identify correctly the people who do not have the condition. If a person is diagnosed as having a condition when the condition is in reality absent, the diagnosis is said to be a false positive (FP), whereas if a diagnostic test is interpreted as negative when the condition is in fact present, the diagnosis is said to be a false negative (FN).

In diagnosing the sex of a baby during pregnancy, an amniocentesis would have higher sensitivity and specificity rates than an ultrasound. Similarly, an ultrasound examination would be expected to have a higher sensitivity and specificity for the diagnosis of intra-uterine growth restriction (IUGR) than abdominal palpation. An ultrasound would be more likely to diagnose (sensitivity) or exclude (specificity) IUGR correctly.

Box 5.2   The Sex of the Baby

The ultrasound on Mrs X indicated that the baby she carried was a boy. A few months later, Mrs X delivered a baby girl. Clearly this baby had two X chromosomes all along (her condition), yet the test (ultrasound) stated that this baby was a boy.

Whereas sensitivity and specificity refer to the ability of the test to identify the presence or the absence of the condition, the predictive value of a test refers to the proportion of accurate tests for either positive or negative test results. The predictive value of a positive test (PV+) refers to the proportion of accurate positive tests given all the positive tests results. The same principle applies for the predictive negative value of a test (PV–).

Low et al. (1999) undertook a study to examine the predictive value of electronic fetal monitoring for intrapartum fetal asphyxia with metabolic acidosis. One of the issues which prompted this research was the number of times that intrapartum fetal asphyxia was thought to be present when it was absent – in other words, the high false positive rate of intrapartum intrauterine asphyxia. It is easy to recall instances when electronic fetal monitoring (EFM) appeared to suggest intrapartum asphyxia in a baby with excellent Apgar scores. The aim of the study was to determine the sensitivity, specificity and prediction of outcomes of four different patterns of EFM.

The study demonstrated that if absent baseline variability for ≥10 minutes AND late and/or prolonged decelerations are used as the criteria for the diagnosis of asphyxia, 98% of the cases where asphyxia is not present will be correctly identified (TNR), but only 17% of the cases where asphyxia is present (TPR) will be picked up. On the other hand, of all the positive diagnoses made only 18% will be correct (PV+), which means that 82% of the diagnoses of fetal asphyxia will be incorrect, but where the fetus is thought not to suffer from asphyxia, the diagnosis will be correct in 98.3% (PV–). Using a 20-minutes criteria improved the sensitivity of the test to 46%, but the specificity is reduced and the predictive value of a positive test falls to 8%. Clearly, using these criteria mean that a large proportion of positive diagnoses will be incorrect, but will be associated with an increase in interventions, particularly Caesarean sections.

Information regarding the incidence of fetal compromise or hypoxia in healthy term pregnancies in spontaneous labour is scarce, and there is often no distinction between what is considered normal or pathological, in either term or pre-term pregnancies. For example, Ingemarsson et al. (1993) studied 1041 women admitted after 34 weeks of gestation in the first stage of labour and administered a 20-minute admission cardiotocograph (CTG). The results were concealed from the clinicians managing labour. "Fetal compromise was considered present when subsequent fetal heart changes resulted in a Caesarean section or forceps delivery, or if the baby was depressed (Apgar score less than 7 at 5 minutes) after spontaneous delivery." No distinction was made between pre- and term pregnancies, healthy and pathological pregnancies.

Comparing babies delivered operatively, whether vaginally or abdominally, with babies whose Apgar was lower than 7 at 5 minutes if born spontaneously, does not take into consideration the effects of the mode of birth itself. Despite the poor correlation with fetal acidaemia or a low Apgar score at birth, admission CTG was advocated despite a clear low sensitivity and predictive value (Ingemarsson et al. 1993). This supports research which identifies that knowledge is not necessarily associated with a change in clinical behaviour (Hamm 2000). Indeed, EFM is no longer recommended for the intrapartum care of healthy women suitable for midwifery-led care (National Institute of Clinical Excellence [NICE] 2001; World Health Organization 1996).

It is natural to think that when a diagnostic test is positive, the disease or the condition should indeed be present. However, a better understanding of the concepts of sensitivity and specificity should help healthcare professionals to question the quality of tests and to select appropriate tests, so as to select appropriate tests better, interpret results more critically, and so avoid errors of interpretation and therefore to potential errors of treatment. Information about test reliability is now more generally available, thanks to the computerisation of maternity data. Summarised annual or monthly reports are regularly produced at local, regional or national levels.

DECISION MAKING

Clinical decision making can be simply defined as involving the selection of a specific treatment over another (Haynes de Regt et al. 1986). The first part of the chapter has explored the complex nature of judgement, and quite a lot of attention has been given to the possibility of errors in diagnosis. Although considering the very real possibilities of making errors might at first sight appear depressing, a sound understanding of the possibility of errors should make practitioners wiser when choosing or proposing various options for treatment or care. It obviously follows that errors in diagnosis can lead to errors in treatment.

Clinical decision making is a multi-dimensional activity which is influenced by several aspects, including clinical experience, research evidence and individual preference, as well as available resources (Flemming and Fenton 2001). Clinical experience can be defined as the level of expertise that comes from dealing with similar situations on a number of occasions. Clinical expertise is ". . . the ability to use our clinical skills and past experience to rapidly identify each patient's unique health state and diagnosis, their individual risks and benefits of potential interventions, and their personal values and expectations" (Sackett et al. 2000).

Clinical experience also comes from learning from peers and authoritative figures. But if the answer to the question "Why are we doing x, y or z this way?" is merely "We have always done it this way", then clinical experience may be more a matter of routine than clinical judgement. Midwives should be aware of the influence of their environment on their clinical practice (Kirkham 1999). A recent study of the intrapartum care of healthy nulliparous women in spontaneous labour at term demonstrated wide variations (Mead 2001).

Good decision making first requires the correct framing of the question (Bordley 2001). The second basis of decision making is research evidence and the elucidation of individuals' values or preferences. The latter will include an appreciation of the various trade-offs of the various options (Bordley 2001). Evidence-based practice is ". . . the integration of best research evidence with clinical expertise and patients' values." (Sackett et al. 2000).

Midwives are involved in decision making at many levels. These are often linked to judgements they have made on the status of particular situations; for example, pattern of antenatal care; admission or discharge home of a woman diagnosed to be in very early labour; timing of transfer of care of mother with a breech presentation; testing serum bilirubin of a baby who appears jaundiced on the third day; calling medical aid if labour is not progressing 'normally'; timing of home visits in the post-natal period; and the use of a birthing pool during labour and birth. Decision making is also linked to values that professionals and women attribute to procedures and outcomes.

Pregnant women are often labelled as having either a low- or a high-risk pregnancy. This labelling may have the undesirable effect of making them a subject of medical interest (Skrabanek and McCormick 1992). This classification tends to define the pregnancy as a whole, rather than a particular aspect that may give cause for concern. It is also useful to remember that the classification in either category can be mistaken, and even if the high-risk or abnormal diagnosis was correct, the identified condition may not by itself necessarily cause the patient any harm (Eddy 1984).

DECISION ANALYSIS

Decision analysis provides ". . . a formal analytic framework that is increasingly being applied to the problem of selecting an action in clinical situations in which the optimal choice is not intuitively clear or the judgements of competent physicians differ. These situations often involve complex combinations of uncertainty, values, risks, and benefits, precisely where human judgement may encounter difficulty in reaching an optimal solution and where a decision aid may be useful." (Elstein et al. 1986).

Since decision making is so complex and error-prone, models have been devised to guide good decisions. These models aim to make decisions more objective and quantifiable. Base rate information can be used to calculate the probability of a particular outcome. The best known of these models is the Bayesian method or Bayes' theorem. This was discussed in more detail in Chapter 4, but the basics are outlined here for ease of reference. Base rate information can be used to calculate the probability of a particular outcome. Three types of evidence are used:

* The prior probability of the existence of a condition that can be based on experiential (Rayburn and Zhang 2002) or epidemiological studies (Haynes de Regt et al. 1986, Spiegelhalter et al. 1999). This is similar to the prevalence of a condition in the population under examination.
* The conditional probability of a positive test given the presence of the condition. This is similar to the sensitivity of a test.
* The posterior probability which combines the prior probability and the conditional probability.

This can be expressed as:

$$P(\text{disease} \mid \text{findings}) = \frac{P(\text{findings} \mid \text{disease}) \times P(\text{disease})}{P(\text{findings})}$$

This type of analysis could be used to calculate the risks of particular problems, for example the risk of fetal hypoxia or admission to a special care baby unit (SCBU) given the presence of meconium-stained liquor, in an otherwise normal pregnancy and labour.

If levels of risk are to be established, it is important to report figures for such eventualities for healthy women with normal pregnancies in spontaneous labour at term. Although the data are theoretically available where maternity units collect computerised information, the level of descriptive detail that would be necessary to establish a Bayesian model equation is not usually readily available to midwives or obstetrician in delivery suites. This shortcoming is not limited to midwifery and obstetrics. If diagnoses or prognoses are to be improved, even in the face of complex individual health problems, then probabilistic models that match individual data against epidemiological data need to be developed. With the increased use of computer facilities and specific computer simulation programs, decisions could also be tailored to individual patients (Delaney et al. 1999).

PRINCIPLES OF DECISION ANALYSIS

Decision analysis combines probabilities of the potential outcomes with the values that these outcomes can have for an individual or groups. This process of decision making can therefore be said to be 'prescriptive', since it is presumed that the outcome that combines the best chances and the best values for the outcomes would be the decision of choice.

Bordley (2001) reviewed the six conditions necessary for prescriptive decision making:

- The problem must be correctly defined.
- Values, preferences, and trade-offs must be clearly articulated.
- A wide range of creative solutions to the problem must be explored.
- Credible relevant data must be used for evaluating these alternatives.
- Logically correct reasoning must be used to evaluated alternatives.
- All the proper stakeholders need to be involved to ensure a commitment to acting on the results of the analysis.

Box 5.3 gives an example of a defined problem and the choices and potential outcomes that may result from a decision.

Numerical values are ascribed to each choice. Individuals can weight each choice according to their own preferences. This means that decisions are personal and pertinent to individuals. In decision analysis, decision trees are drawn to represent choices and outcomes. Individual weightings are added to these decision trees, in order to guide the decision-making process.

The example of the decision to study or not to study can be used to demonstrate how

---

Box 5.3 To Study or Not to Study

- The problem is clearly defined: an exam is looming.
- Values, preferences, trade-offs are clearly articulated: it is important to pass this exam, but studying is a bind. On the other hand, a failure will mean that holiday will be spent studying for the re-sits.
- Creative solutions are not really catered for in the university regulations...
- Credible relevant data: success tends to follow study and failure tends to follow absence of study.
- Correct reasoning follows previous item.
- Stakeholders – student, lecturer, exam board and professional body, friends – a pass will mean progression and possibly registration. Systematic failure will mean eventually seeking an alternative type of occupation. On the other hand, there is that holiday with friends.

---

decisions can vary for Student A or Student B. The previous experience of the two students shows that they achieve a 90% pass rate if they study, but only a 40% pass rate if they do not study. This means that if these two students study, they have 90% chance of a pass and a good holiday, but if they do not study, they only have a 60% chance of a fail and a holiday spent studying. At first, the choice might seem obvious – study and get a good holiday. But individual preferences play a part in the decision to study or not to study. Individuals are asked to provide a rating for the various outcomes, usually measured between 0 and 100. These 'values' are personal to each individual, and are included in a decision analysis to make the choice specifically pertinent to individuals. This is called 'maximising utilities'.

In this example of Students A and B, previous experience suggest the following results (Figure 5.1).

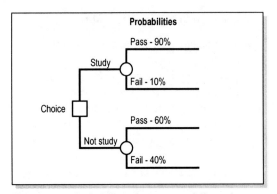

Figure 5.1 Probability of success or failure given study or no study.

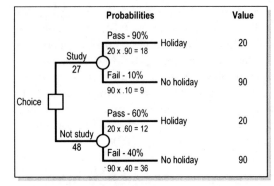

Figure 5.3 Maximised utilities – Student B.

Student A really wants to go on holiday, so the value that is given to the holiday is 100 compared to only 20 for having to stay at home and study again. Those values remain the same whether this student studies initially or does not.

The choice (represented by a □) needs to take into consideration the probabilities of the outcomes (represented by a ○) and the values given to those outcomes. The values, or expected utilities, take probabilities of the various outcomes given the various choices into consideration, but also take into consideration personal preferences, thereby making the choice personal.

Student A provides the following values for the outcomes: holiday 100 and no holiday 20 (Figure 5.2); Student B cannot stand holidays because they always mean family torture, and so attributes the following values: holiday 20 and no holiday 90 (Figure 5.3).

The utility of the holiday is multiplied by the probabilities of passing and the utility of not having a holiday is multiplied by the probabilities of failing. This model is logical and rational. The rule means that the higher utility is the one that ought to be chosen.

So for Student A, the total utilities for the study option are $(100 \times 0.90) + (20 \times 0.10)$ or $(90 + 2) = 92$; for the no study option the total utilities are $(100 \times 0.60) + (20 \times 0.40)$ or $(60 + 8) = 68$. As 92 is greater than 68, the rational choice for Student A is therefore the option to study.

For Student B, the utilities are quite different and the total utilities score 27 for the study option and 48 for the no study option. In this case, the rational choice for Student B would be not to study.

This example is simple to the point of being simplistic, as clearly there are more outcomes to consider than simply having a free or a studying holiday, but it demonstrates the point.

Clinical situations can be far more complex, but the principles remain the same: construct a mathematical model (decision tree) that details the various options and their potential consequences and assign probabilities and values to the various outcomes. Finally, once the expected utilities have been calculated, with the highest being the optimal one, examine how sensitive the decision is given variations within a normal range for both probabilities and values (Doubilet and McNeil 1985).

The next example represents an example of a decision that could be made by a first-time mother, given the analysis of onset of labour and

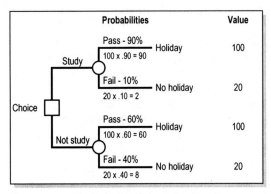

Figure 5.2 Maximised utilities – Student A.

mode of birth. This example is presented in several steps. First, the evidence base is presented. The evidence is then used to form a decision tree. The figures used here are extracted from a database of 7381 healthy women at term. Most of these women (7311) accessed the maternity services through the NHS, and a few (70) paid for private care. The NHS and private sector data demonstrated differences in methods of onset of labour (see Table 5.1). The differences observed were statistically significant ($\chi^2 = 25.170$, df 2, $p < 0.001$).

Induction of labour was associated with an increased risk of operative vaginal deliveries and emergency Caesarean sections (Table 5.2). These differences were also statistically significant ($\chi^2 = 152.744$, df 2, $p < 0.001$).

Mothers who experienced NHS care had a higher rate of spontaneous birth than women receiving private maternity care, whether the onset of labour was spontaneous or induced (see Table 5.3), but these differences did not reach a significance level (spontaneous onset $\chi^2 = 4.623$, df 2, $p = 0.099$; induction $\chi^2 = 2.939$, df 2, $p = 0.230$).

Should a mother select the NHS or private option? The various modes of birth have been reproduced in Figure 5.4 according to the methods of onset of labour and types of client category. These values of three mothers (Mother A, Mother B and Mother C) have then been incorporated to calculate the maximised

Table 5.1 Patient Category and Method of Onset of Labour

		Patient Category		
		Normal	Private	Total
Induction	n	1314	23	1337
	%	18.0	32.9	18.1
Elective CS	n	312	9	321
	%	4.3	12.9	4.3
Spontaneous	n	5685	38	5723
	%	77.8	54.3	77.5
	n	7311	70	7381
	%	100.0	100.0	100.0

Table 5.2 Method of Delivery by Onset of Labour. FD & VE = Forceps Delivery and Vacuum Extraction

		Onset of Labour		
		Induction	Sponta-neous	Total
Normal	n	636	3598	4234
	%	47.8	64.0	60.9
FD & VE	n	414	1423	1837
	%	31.1	25.3	26.4
Emerg CS	n	280	597	877
	%	21.1	10.6	12.6
Total	n	1330	5618	6948
	%	100.0	100.0	100.0

utilities and the three mothers in their choice of NHS versus private maternity care. This is illustrated in the following scenario. Mother A, Mother B and Mother C all have distinct values:

* Mother A places a high value on normal delivery.
* Mother B prefers a normal delivery, but also places a high value on Caesarean section.
* Mother C prefers a Caesarean section.

Their values have been multiplied by the chances of each outcome, and then totalled to produce the score for the NHS or the private options. Mother A and Mother B should be advised to opt for the NHS, but Mother C has such a high value for a Caesarean section, whether elective or emergency that her optimum choice should be the private option (see Figure 5.4).

A number of clinical alternatives can serve as examples: antenatal screening or diagnostic tests, including amniocentesis and/or ultrasound, use of CTGs or epidural during spontaneous labour for healthy women at term of a healthy pregnancy, screening babies for phenylketonuria, elective Caesarean section on demand, immunisation of children, etc. Indeed, personal choices have given rise to debate, often because of conflicting values. Little benefit is gained from drawing a decision

Table 5.3 Method of Delivery by Onset of Labour and Provider of Care

Onset of Labour				Care Category		
				NHS	Private	Total
Induction	Method delivery	Normal	n	629	7	636
			%	48.1	30.4	47.8
		FD & VE	n	405	9	414
			%	31.0	39.1	31.1
		Emerg CS	n	273	7	280
			%	20.9	30.4	21.1
	Total		n	1307	23	1330
			%	100.0	100.0	100.0
Spontaneous	Method delivery	Normal	n	3580	18	3598
			%	64.2	47.4	64.0
		FD & VE	n	1409	14	1423
			%	25.3	36.8	25.3
		Emerg	n	591	6	597
			%	10.6	15.8	10.6
	Total		n	5580	38	5618
			%	100.0	100.0	100.0

tree for the advantages or disadvantages of a particular set of choices when the individuals would never consider one of the options and would give a value of zero to that option. In that case, the calculation of the expected utilities would always produce a score of zero for that option, and an alternative option would always be the rational choice. However, where the best choice is not evident, it can be useful to combine options with the values of the individuals concerned.

For each of these examples, alternative options can be identified: to measure or not measure a pregnant woman's blood pressure during pregnancy; to have or not to have an antenatal screening or diagnostic test; to monitor fetal health by the use of a CTG or auscultation; to use an epidural or other forms of pain relief; to screen babies for phenylketonuria or not; to opt for an elective Caesarean section or to choose spontaneous labour, etc. Each option will itself be associated with potential outcomes of varying probabilities. Each outcome will have varying degrees of acceptability or value for

the mother and her baby. A classic example of decision analysis is that of the decision to have or not to have an amniocentesis for a 40-year-old woman (Pauker and Pauker 1977).

The concept of decision trees including probabilities and values is quite simple. However, determining probabilities is not necessarily simple. Probabilities can be objectively determined, for example the decision regarding amniocentesis (Flemming and Fenton 2001, Pauker and Pauker 1977). However, it is useful to note that, given the potential usefulness of decision trees, this study remains a classic after more than 25 years, perhaps because no other decision tree specific to maternity care has been published.

COMPLEXITIES AND LIMITATIONS ASSOCIATED WITH DECISION ANALYSIS

The requirement for objectively determined probabilities is one of the main difficulties associated with decision analysis. It requires extensive review of the literature on individuals

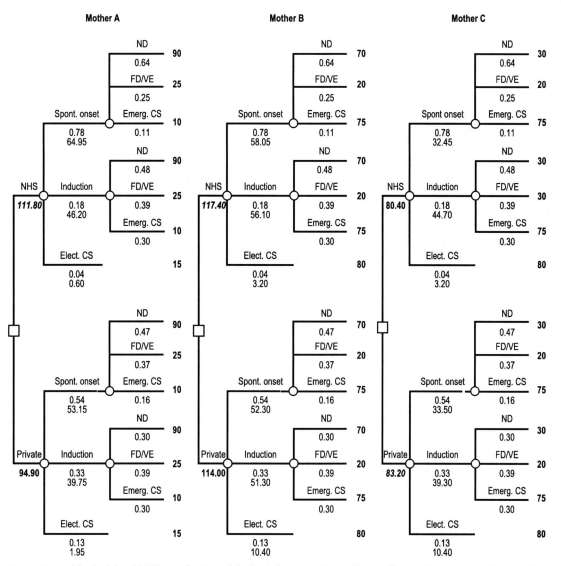

Figure 5.4 Maximising Utilities – Choice of Patient Category According to Onset of Labour and Methods of Delivery – Mother A, Mother B, and Mother C.

similar to the subject under consideration and assumptions that the statistics provided by studies may be applicable in the present situation. Such an approach provides a robust statistical basis, but there is also the danger of arriving at incorrect results where the assumption of cause and effect relationships is doubtful. This probabilistic approach also requires the design of potentially very complex decision trees, if all potential outcomes are to be explored. One alternative to using objectively constructed probabilities is the use of subjective estimation of probabilities. Unfortunately, physicians (Lichenstein et al. 1978) and midwives (Mead 2001), tend to over- or under-estimate the likelihood of particular events (Lichenstein et al. 1978). Furthermore, even when likelihoods are understood, seemingly irrational choices are still made (Hamm 2000).

Another alternative is the design of simplified decision trees that only identify some of the options or some of the outcomes. Such an approach was used to help a couple focus on some of the choices they may have to think about when considering a further pregnancy following the birth of a healthy daughter, and then the birth of a son who died at 18 months from a lethal recessive genetic abnormality. The parents had rejected the possibility of a spontaneous pregnancy because they felt that a 25% risk was too high. A simplified decision tree was drawn identifying three options for consideration, with the understanding that reproductive technologies may have alternatives to offer: (1) no further pregnancy; (2) assisted reproduction with the help of sperm donation; or (3) assisted reproduction with the help of egg donation.

ALTERNATIVE WAYS OF ANALYSING DECISIONS

There is a growing body of evidence, mostly backed by qualitative research, that describes how nurses or midwives make decisions (Haggerty 1996, Levy 1999). This is essentially different from the larger psychology-based literature on medical decision making which is more likely to be quantitative and linked to the search for a more prescriptive line of action (Haynes de Regt et al. 1986, Sackett et al. 2000). In his review of the clinical decision-making theory in nursing, Thompson (1999) explores the cognitive continuum that underpins nursing decision making, from the Bayes' theorem, which requires adherence to strict mathematical rules, to the intuitive stance (Benner and Tanner 1987) already discussed. Thompson (1999) argues that the two approaches are not 'adversaries', but rather the ends of a descriptive to prescriptive continuum.

Midwives have generally not been the subjects of such investigation or analysis, although some research has been published on the heuristics, or rules of thumb, used by midwives in low- or high-complexity standardised scenarios (Cioffi 1997), and in the assessment of fetal stress by 'intrapartal nurses' in the United States (Haggerty 1996). Grounded theory has also been used to describe the processes used by midwives to facilitate maternal choices during pregnancy (Levy 1999). The purpose of these studies was not to identify prescriptive models for optimal choices in the presence of quantified outcomes or elicited personal values, but rather to describe specific patterns of decision making used by midwives.

CONCLUSION

Mathematical theories of decision making, such as the Bayesian model, assume that decisions are made along the lines of a rational procedure which assumes optimal strategies. It has been suggested that individuals tend to follow Bayesian rules in estimating probabilities, but fail to appreciate the full impact of the evidence presented and in consequence tend to act conservatively (Edwards 1968, cited in Rayburn and Zhang 2002). However, further studies have demonstrated that human beings – including doctors – were rather poor at using Bayesian models when confronted with a positive diagnostic test as they tended to ignore prior probabilities and false-positives (DeGowin and DeGowin 1969; Kahneman et al. 1982). A high sensitivity or true positive rate (i.e. the ability of a test to be positive in the presence of a disease) cannot reveal whether the condition is likely or very likely unless it is accompanied by a low false-positive rate (i.e. the rate of positive diagnosis in the absence of the disease).

The improvement of the limited ability of medical practitioners – and by extrapolation midwives – to integrate these two concepts when estimating the likelihood of a condition has been targeted by some researchers, but the discrepancies remain between the results that could be obtained via Bayes' theorem and clinical judgement (Dawes 1988; DeGowin and DeGowin 1969; Haynes de Regt et al. 1986).

The application of probabilities can be supplemented by the determination of the subjective values of the potential outcomes for individuals, thereby maximising personal choices. Since the importance of patient satisfaction and informed choice and consent is now recognised and accepted, subjective expected utilities could, in principle, form the basis for patient information and choice (O'Connor et al. 1999; Scally and Donaldson 1998). The elicitation of quantified utilities is challenging and as yet poorly developed in health research or practice (Spiegelhalter et al. 1999).

Computerised models of decision seem to have certain advantages but have not yet been integrated into practice. Extensive research would first have to be undertaken to enable the determination of prior and posterior probabilities for the application of a Bayesian approach to the maternity services. Indeed, in their appraisal of the required developments in the context of the health technology assessments, Spiegelhalter et al. (1999) recommend: (1) an extended set of case studies showing practical aspects of the Bayesian approach, in particular for prediction and handling multiple sub-studies, in which mathematical details are minimised; (2) the development of standards for the performance and reporting of Bayesian analyses; and (3) the development and dissemination of software for Bayesian analysis, preferably as part of existing programs.

On a daily basis, midwives are confronted with decisions about the normality of a pregnancy, labour, puerperium and neonate. Several aspects need to be considered: (1) a more realistic awareness of our ability to make errors; (2) a more realistic awareness of base line probabilities so that midwives' perception of risks are more accurate; (3) tools that midwives could use to assess risks more accurately, e.g. Bayes' theorem; and (4) tools that midwives could use to measure the risks of various options, whilst taking account of individual preferences.

A more accurate probabilistic approach would allow women to clearly identify the outcomes to be considered before choices can be made. It would also enable midwives, GPs and obstetricians to construct basic decision trees based on their practice and outcomes. It could also enable practitioners to be more aware of the potential advantages and disadvantages of various practices.

KEY POINTS FOR BEST PRACTICE

- To be human is to err! We make mistakes; indeed, we make lots and lots of mistakes. Even 'very good' practitioners make mistakes.

- Mistakes can occur when making decisions about diagnosis and/or treatment.

- Human beings cannot juggle too much information at once, yet complex decisions require the evaluation of complex information.

- Intuition – the ability to reach sound conclusions with minimal evidence – is fraught with limitation.

- Sound judgement needs to consider concepts such as incidence or prevalence, sensitivity and specificity, predictive value of a positive or negative diagnosis.

- Alternative approaches to judgement, for example normative decision approaches such as Bayes' theorem, can improve the quality of judgement and reduce the risk of errors.

- Decision making needs to involve a sound understanding of alternatives, and should also include a weighting of the values of the probable alternative outcomes to maximise the quality of choices.

References

Barrett J, Jarvis G, Macdonald H, et al. 1990 Inconsistencies in clinical decisions in obstetrics. The Lancet 336(8714): 549.

Bell D, Raiffa H and Tversky A (eds) 1988 Decision Making: Descriptive, Normative and Prescriptive Interactions, Cambridge University Press, Cambridge.

Benner P 1984 From novice to expert, excellence and power in clinical nursing practice, 1. Addison-Wesley Publishing Company, Nursing Division, London.

Benner P, Tanner C 1987 Clinical judgement: how expert nurses use intuition. American Journal of Nursing 87(1): 23–31.

Berlin S, Marsh J 1993 Informing Practice Decisions. Macmillan Publishing Company, New York.

Bordley R 2001 Naturalistic decision making and prescriptive decision theory. Journal of Behavioral Decision Making 14(5): 355–357.

Bursztajn H, Gutheil TG, Hamm RM, et al. 1988 Parens patriae considerations in the commitment process. The Psychiatric Quarterly 59(3): 165–181.

Cioffi J 1997 Heuristics, servants to intuition, in clinical decision-making. Journal of Advanced Nursing 26(1): 203–208.

Confidential Enquiry into Stillbirths and Deaths in Infancy 2001 8th Annual Report, Maternal and Child Health Research Consortium, London.

Dawes R 1988 Rational Choice in an Uncertain World. Harcourt Brace Jovanovich, New York

DeGowin E, DeGowin R 1969 Bedside Diagnostic Examination, 2nd edition. Macmillan, London.

Delaney B, Fitzmaurice D, Riaz A, et al. 1999 Can computerised decision support systems deliver improved quality in primary care? British Medical Journal 319(7220): 1281–1283.

de Tombal F 1988. Computer-aided diagnosis of acute abdominal pain; the British experience.

In: Dowie J, Elstein A (eds), Professional Judgment, a Reader in Clinical Decision Making. Cambridge University Press, Vol. 1, pp. 190–199.

Doubilet P, McNeil B 1985 In: Dowie J, Elstein A (eds), Professional Judgment, a Reader in Clinical Decision Making. Cambridge University Press.

Eddy D 1984 Variations in physician practice: the role of uncertainty. Health Affairs 3(2): 74–89.

Elstein A, Shulman L, Sprafka S 1978 Medical Problem Solving, an Analysis of Clinical Reasoning. Harvard University Press, Cambridge, Massachusetts.

Elstein AS, Holzman GB, Ravitch MM, et al. 1986 Comparisons of physicians' decisions regarding estrogen replacement therapy for menopausal women and decisions derived from a decision analytic model. American Journal of Medicine 80(2): 246–258.

Eraker S, Politser P 1982 How decisions are reached: physician and patient. Annals of Internal Medicine 97(2): 262–268.

Farmer R, Miller D, Lawrenson R 1996 Epidemiology and Public Health Medicine. Blackwell Science, Oxford.

Flemming K, Fenton M 2001 Making sense of research evidence to inform decision making. In: Thompson P, Dowding D (eds), Clinical Decision Making and Judgement in Nursing. Baillière Tindall, Edinburgh.

Haggerty L 1996 Assessment parameters and indicators in expert intrapartal nursing decisions. Journal of Obstetric, Gynecological and Neonatal Nursing 25(6): 491–499.

Hamm R 2000 Implications of physician illness scripts for the movement for rational decision making. Online. Available: http://www.fammed.ouhsc.edu/robhamm/SMDMnntthreshold/index.htm. Last accessed 29.11.03.

Haynes de Regt R, Minkoff H, Feldman J, et al. 1986 Relation of private or clinic care to the cesarean birth rate. New England Journal of Medicine 315(10): 619–624.

Ingemarsson I, Ingemarsson E, Spencer J 1993 Fetal Heart Rate Monitoring, a practical guide. Oxford University Press, Oxford.

Johnson D 1955 The Psychology of Thought and Judgment. Harper & Row, New York.

Kahneman D, Slovic P, Tversky A 1982 Judgment Under Uncertainty: Heuristics and Biases. Cambridge University Press, Cambridge.

Lichenstein S, Slovic P, Fischhoff B, Layman M, Coombes B 1978 Judged frequency of lethal events. Journal of Experimental Psychology: Human Learning and Memory 4: 551–578.

Katz J 1988 Why doctors don't disclose uncertainty. In: Dowie J, Elstein A (eds), Professional Judgement. Cambridge University Press, Cambridge.

Kirkham M 1999 The culture of midwifery in the National Health Service in England. Journal of Advanced Nursing 30(3): 732–739.

Kirwan J, Chaput de Saintonge D, Joyce C, et al. 1983 Clinical judgment in rheumatoid arthritis. II. Judging 'current disease activity' in clinical practice. Annals of the Rheumatic Diseases 42(6): 686–694.

Kozielecki J 1981 Psychological Decision Theory. PWN-Polish Scientific Publishers, Warsaw.

Levy V 1999 Protective steering: a grounded theory study of the processes by which midwives facilitate informed choices during pregnancy. Journal of Advanced Nursing 29(1): 104–112.

Lewis G, Drife J 2001 Why Mothers Die 1997-1999. The Confidential Enquiries into Maternal Deaths in the UK. The Stationery Office, London.

Lewis G, Drife J 2004 Confidential Enquiry into Maternal and Child Health; Why Mothers Die 2000–2002. Sixth Report of the Confidential Enquiries into Maternal Deaths in the UK. RCOG Press, London.

Low JA, Victory R, Derrick EJ 1999 Predictive value of electronic fetal monitoring for intrapartum fetal asphyxia with metabolic acidosis. Obstetrics and Gynaecology 93: 285–291.

McCaughan D 2002 What decisions do nurses make? In: Thompson C, Dowding D (eds), Clinical Decision Making and Judgement in Nursing. Churchill Livingstone, London.

Mead M 2001 Decision making by midwives in the intrapartum care of women suitable for full midwifery care: processes and influences 2001. Unpublished PhD thesis. University of Hertfordshire.

NICE 2001 The use and interpretation of cardiotocography in intrapartum fetal surveillance (Guideline C). NHS, London.

O'Connor A, Rostom A, Fiset V, et al. 1999 Decision aids for patients facing health treatment or screening decisions: a systematic review. British Medical Journal 319: 731–734.

Pauker S, Pauker S 1977 Prenatal diagnosis; a directive approach to genetic counselling using decision analysis. The Yale Journal of Biology and Medicine 50: 275–289.

Peschel R, Peschel E 1990 The statistical spectre we live with. British Medical Journal 300: 1145.

Rayburn W, Zhang J 2002 rising rates of labor induction: present concerns and future strategies. Obstetrics and Gynecology 100(1): 164–167.

Sackett D, Strauss S, Richardson W, et al. 2000 Evidence-based Medicine: How to Practice and Teach EBM, 2nd edition. Churchill Livingstone, London.

Scally G, Donaldson L 1998 Clinical governance and the drive for quality improvement in the new NHS in England. British Medical Journal 317: 61–65.

Schrader B, Fischer D 1987 Using intuitive knowledge in the neonatal intensive care nursery. Holistic Nursing Practice 1(3): 45–51.

Skrabanek P, McCormick J 1992 Follies and Fallacies in Medicine, 2. The Tarragon Press, Chippenham.

Snyder M 1993 Critical thinking: a foundation for consumer-focused care. The Journal of Continuing Education in Nursing 24(5): 206–210.

Spiegelhalter D, Myles J, Jones D, et al. 1999 An introduction to bayesian methods in health technology assessment. British Medical Journal 319: 508–512.

Thompson C 1999 A conceptual treadmill: the need for 'middle ground' in clinical decision making theory in nursing. Journal of Advanced Nursing 30(5): 1222–1229.

Thornton J 1990 Analysis of probability and measurement of values. Baillière's Clinical Obstetrics and Gynaecology 4(4): 867–884.

Tversky A, Kahneman D 1974 Judgment under uncertainty: Heuristics and biases.In: Kahneman D, Slovic P, Tversky A (eds), Judgment under Uncertainty: Heuristics and Biases. Cambridge University Press, Cambridge, Vol. 3, p. 20.

Weed L, Weed L 1999 Opening the black box of clinical judgment – an overview. British Medical Journal 319: 1279.

Weingart S, Wilson R, Gibberd R, et al. 2000 Epidemiology of medical error. British Medical Journal 320: 774–777.

Wescott M 1968 Toward a Contemporary Psychology of Intuition. Holt, Rinehart & Winston, New York.

World Health Organization 1996 Care in Normal birth: A Practical Guide. WHO, Geneva.

Further Reading

Books

French S, Smith J 1997 The Practice of Bayesian Analysis. Arnold, London.

Gelman A 1995 Bayesian Data Analysis. Chapman & Hall, London.

Gigerenzer G, Todd PM, and ABC Research Group 1999 Simple Heuristics That Make Us Smart. Oxford University Press, New York.

Iversen GR 1984 Bayesian Statistical Inference. Sage, Beverly Hills, London.

Jensen F 1996 An Introduction to Bayesian Networks. UCL Press, London.

Kammen DM, Hassenzahl DM 1999 Should We Risk It?: Exploring Environmental, Health, and Technological Problem Solving. Princeton University Press, Princeton, NJ.

Lee PM 2004 Bayesian Statistics: An Introduction. Arnold, London.

Maritz JS, Lwin T 1989 Empirical Bayes Methods. Chapman & Hall, London.

Martin JJ 1967 Bayesian Decision Problems and Markov Chains. Wiley, Chichester.

Morton A 1997 A Guide through the Theory of Knowledge. Blackwell, Oxford.

Parmigiani G 2002 Modeling in Medical Decision Making: A Bayesian Approach. Wiley, Chichester.

Press SJ 1989 Bayesian Statistics: Principles, Models, and Applications. John Wiley, Chichester.

Ríos S, Ríos Insua D, Ríos-Insua S 1994 Decision Theory and Decision Analysis: Trends and Challenges. Kluwer Academic, Boston, London.

Rosenkrantz RD 1977 Inference, Method, and Decision: Towards a Bayesian Philosophy of Science. D. Reidel Publishing

Co., Dordrecht, Holland, Boston.

Sklar L 1999 Bayesian and Non-Inductive Strategies. Routledge.

Spiegelhalter DJ, Abrams KR, Myles JP 2004 Bayesian Approaches to Clinical Trials and Health-Care Evaluation. John Wiley & Sons, Chichester.

Spiegelhalter DJ and National Coordinating Centre for Health Technology Assessment 2000 Bayesian Methods in Health Technology Assessment: A Review. NCCHTA.

Stevens A 2000 The Advanced Handbook of Methods in Evidence Based Healthcare. Sage, London.

Journals

Bates D, Cohen M, Leape L, Overhage J, Shabot M, Sheridan T 2001 reducing the frequency of errors in medicine using information technology. Journal of the American Medical Informatics Association 8(4): 299–308.

Briggs A 2000 Handling uncertainty in cost-effectiveness models. Pharmacoeconomics 17(5): 479–500.

Buckingham CD, Adams A 2000 Classifying clinical decision making: a unifying approach. Journal of Advanced Nursing 32(4): 981–989.

Buckingham CD, Adams A 2000 Classifying clinical decision making: interpreting nursing intuition, heuristics and medical diagnosis. Journal of Advanced Nursing 32(4): 990–998.

Cartmill RS, Thornton JG 1992 Effect of presentation of partogram information on obstetric decision-making. The Lancet 339(8808): 1520–1522.

Handfield B, Bell R 1995 Do childbirth classes influence decision making about labor and postpartum issues? Birth 22(3): 153–160.

Kaushal R, Barker K, Bates D 2001 How can information technology improve patient safety and reduce medication errors in children's health care? Archives of Pediatrics and Adolescent Medicine 155(9): 1002–1007.

Lipman T, Price D 2000 Decision making, evidence, audit, and education: case study of antibiotic prescribing in general practice. British Medical Journal 320(7242): 1114–1148.

O'Connor A, Stacey D, Rovner D, Holmes-Rovner M, Tetroe J, Llewellyn-Thomas H, Entwistle V, Rostom A, Fiset V, Barry M, Jones J 2001 Decision aids for people facing health treatment or screening decisions. Cochrane Database of Systematic Reviews(3): CD001431.

O'Connell RL, Gebski VJ, Keech AC 2004 Making sense of trial results: outcomes and estimation. Medical Journal of Australia 180(3): 128–130.

Shorten A, Chamberlain M, Shorten B, Kariminia A 2004 Making choices for childbirth: development and testing of a decision-aid for women who have experienced previous caesarean. Patient Education and Counselling 52(3): 307–313.

Sommer PA, Norr K, Roberts J 2000 Clinical decision-making regarding intravenous hydration in normal labor in a birth center setting. Journal of Midwifery and Women's Health 45(2): 114–121.

Steward M 2001 Whose Evidence Counts? An exploration of health professionals' perceptions of evidence-based practice, focusing on the maternity services. Midwifery 17(4): 279–288.

Stotland NE, Lipschitz LS, Caughey AB 2002 Delivery strategies for women with a previous classic cesarean delivery: a decision analysis. American Journal of Obstetrics and Gynecology 187(5): 1203–1208.

Thornton H, Edwards A, Elwyn G 2003 evolving the multiple roles of 'patients' in health-care research: reflections after involvement in a trial of shared decision-making. Health Expect 6(3): 189–197.

Todd M 2002 Organisational Culture and Decision Making. Managing and Implementing Decisions in Health Care. A Young and M Cooke. London, Baillière Tindall in Association with RCN.

Vandevusse L 1999 Decision making in analyses of women's birth stories. Birth 26(1): 43–50.

Websites

Some examples include:

National Electronic Library for Health http://www.nelh.nhs.uk/

The Bugs Project http://www.mrcbsu.cam.ac.uk/bugs/welcome.shtml

Centre for Health Evidence - University of Alberta http://www.cche.net/che/home.asp

Centre for Reviews and Dissemination - University of York http://www.york.ac.uk/inst/crd/

Robert Hamm web site http://www.fammed.ouhsc.edu/robhamm/

How to use the evidence: assessment and application of scientific evidence

http://www.health.gov.au/nhmrc/publications/pdf/cp69.pdf

Email Lists

For a list of e-mail lists of interest for medicine and health: http://www.jiscmail.ac.uk/mailinglists/category/Medicine_&_Health.htm including amongst many others:

- Centre for Evidence based medicine http:// www.jiscmail.ac.uk/lists/CEBM-MEMBERS.html
- Critical Appraisal Skills http://www.jiscmail.ac.uk/lists/CRITICAL-APPRAISAL-SKILLS.html
- Evidence Based Health http://www.jiscmail.ac.uk/lists/EVIDENCE-BASED-HEALTH.html
- Midwifery Research http://www.jiscmail.ac.uk/lists/MIDWIFERY-RESEARCH.html

Chapter 6

Developing Clinical Judgements

Sally Marchant

THE DEVELOPMENT OF PROFESSIONAL JUDGEMENT AND ITS CONTRIBUTION TO DECISION MAKING

Many readers familiar with the way of life in the United Kingdom will be aware of the following few words that have become a contemporary catchphrase over the past couple of years – "Is that your final answer?" This is from a popular game/quiz show called 'Who wants to be a millionaire?' (Celador 2003). Interested contestants put themselves forward, and the one selected has to choose the correct answer from a list of four possible answers in order to continue in the game, winning variable amounts of money in the process up to the goal of one million pounds. The interest in this game is the process by which the contestant makes judgements and decisions. This is not wildly different from the overall framework used in any process that involves the examination of new and/or existing knowledge vetted against intrinsic values, attitudes or beliefs and utilised by the ethical or moral baseline of the individual. Taking the millionaire example further; although it seems as though the contestant is making these judgements or decision on his or her own behalf, in all cases the outcome is being witnessed by a huge number of people (some present but most hidden), and for many contestants the outcome will have a significant effect on their friends and families. So what drives this process? Can it actually be defined or explained as a single concept, or is it more a complex interaction of various philosophical entities that happen, by virtue of their single aim – to resolve a quandary or problem?

Reviewing the literature about professional judgement and decision making reveals a level of academic debate and discourse that is not particularly cogent with the very practice it is designed to support. The philosophical debate is not easily accessible to the emerging health-care professional who will be required to make judgements and decisions from the moment they engage in any form of health and/or social care of others. There appears to be more publications about making decisions than judgements, but overall there are several ideo-logical or theoretical models. These relate more to nursing than midwifery care but they describe the process of clinical judgement, diagnosis and decision making and explain the use of these by clinicians in moving forward from mere attendant and observer, to analyst and initiator (Benner 1982, Buckingham and Adams 2000a, Thompson et al. 2001, Thompson 2001). The main theories relate to the **hypo-thetico-deductive process** based on the assess-ment of probability. The alternative is described as a **reasoning and intuitive approach** where what is observed, overtly and covertly (intu-itively) is added into the equation along with existing knowledge about that individual or the circumstances surrounding an event (Barker 2001, Buckingham and Adams 2000a, Effken 2001, King and Appleton 1997, Thompson 2001).

So what is judgement, and what pressure is placed on judgement when this relates to judgements taken by professionals rather than 'the common man'? A famous judgement made over 40 years ago, defined actions that can be expected of the 'expert' as opposed to those that might be taken by someone without that level of knowledge. This resulted in the **Bolam Standard** for Clinical Negligence claims (Bolam v. Friern Hospital Management Committee 1957). The judgement defined the explicit responsibility of taking action in line with that expectation. This is important when considering negligence, where the notion of what denotes negligence is linked to the stan-dard of care expected from someone with skills and knowledge (the professional) against someone without this. Although there have been judgements that have clarified this approach (Dimond 2001), this has been the mainstay for the process of judgement within the clinical setting and against which profes-sional conduct is assessed (Benner 1982, Pyne 1992, Nursing and Midwifery Council [NMC] 2004a). Whether the 'Bolam test' is still relevant to current healthcare practices is now being questioned alongside judgement from another court case (Bolitho v. City & Hackney Health Authority 1997) that defines still further the difference between the status of the profes-sional and then the expert (Dimond 2001, Symon 1999, Tingle 2002). The **Bolitho princi-ple** states that actions must have a logical basis, although some practice conventions may not appear to have this. Nevertheless, these are important areas for how judgements of the practice and conduct of professionals have been and will continue to be made.

From making the judgement, there is then the decision – arguably these are inextricably linked as part of a continuum or cycle of care in the clinical environment where one process may initiate another and then be reassessed so that the whole process starts again (Buckingham and Adams 2000a, Thompson 1999, 2001). Where there is confu-sion about the different but also interactive parts in this circle there is also likely to be uncertainty and a negative effect on outcomes in the healthcare setting (Buckingham and Adams 2000b). This chapter explores these factors more widely than the clinical field to incorporate education and management. As these are all components of the eventual care provided by healthcare professionals, it appears logical to include them.

The concept of professional judgement is that it should precede action taken as a result of a decision arising from that judgement (Thompson 1999, Thompson et al. 2001, Buckingham and Adams 2000a). Even in extreme emergency situations, there is still a process of rapid assessment, summing up and judgement in order to make a decision and take action. This is the process, but the factors that are used within the process are critical to the ultimate veracity of the judgement and eventual outcome.

There is a significant contribution in the literature on this subject from the nursing and medical disciplines. This is to be expected where the burden of professional diagnosis and care management is accepted as being the responsibility, jointly or severally, of these two disciplines and where the concept of sharing decisions with patients is an emerging philosophy rather than the accepted approach to care (Charles et al. 1997, Friend 1995, Trede and Higgs 2003).

With regard to midwifery, the relationship of healthcare professional and woman is commonly argued as being different from that of healthcare professional (carer) and patient (involuntary recipient of care). Both in midwifery and to some extent in obstetric care, the acknowledged difference is that the majority of women are not suffering from a state of ill health in their pregnancy but are rather more enjoying the fulfilment of their womanhood (Kitzinger 1997), and that being pregnant is a natural and normal event (Page 2003). This concept of wellness as opposed to illness is seen as being pivotal to how women are then involved in the decision-making process. The health professional aims to be an advisor and supporter, particularly by helping women access information for themselves. Where this occurs, women can then exercise greater freedom of personal choice and can be voluntary recipients of care, where this is appropriate (Department of Health [DoH] 1993, Friend 1995, Harding 2000). The presence of health-related complications for either the woman or fetus may alter this relationship, and the woman may become more dependent on the healthcare professional's skills and knowledge. This may result in a change of balance in the relationship so that the healthcare professional is placed in a situation where there is an expectation that judgements and decisions will be made on behalf of the woman and maybe the fetus within the key ethical principles

(Barwise 1998, Gillon 1994, Kirkham et al. 2002) (see also Chapter 7).

DEFINING JUDGEMENT

It is not always helpful to have a simple definition, as this can be a rather narrow concept where this is a complex concept that cannot be encompassed as a single entity. The verb 'to judge' can also be linked with other words, for example, pre-judging, mis-judging and judgmental. All of these words could be viewed as evoking negative values to the process as they link with a much wider ethical and cultural framework where judgement and punishment or the receipt of 'just desserts' (good or bad) are brought to mind. This in turn may explain its attraction for the many philosophical perspectives presented within the literature in an attempt to explore how something occurs, rather than just describing what it is. How judgements are taken are explained as a continuum of comparative phases that involve the process of analysis of existing information, the presumption of future events and the consolidation of these to resolution of the enquiry. For nursing and midwifery, there is contradiction with the more medical model where, for non-medical practitioners, there is the inclusion and some reliance on intuition. This is explained as an understanding of a situation without necessarily having any justification or explanation for this (Benner and Tanner 1987) (see Chapter 2).

From the perspective of this chapter, an awareness of the philosophical framework that is thought to support how people make judgements in clinical practice is important, bearing in mind that as far as individual women, their baby and their family is concerned, it is more likely to be the impact of the overall process that is of importance to them. Therefore, where these theories can explain why a particular course of action might have been taken, this may be helpful to both carer and recipient to reach an understanding of how the judgement came to be, sometimes over-riding the eventual outcome (Van de Vusse 1999, Vandenbussche et al. 1999). It is also helpful to identify a course of action in which the outcome was either negative or positive and reflect on the rationale of the judgement made at the time, acknowledging the benefit of hindsight but not judging the effectiveness on the basis of this.

APPROACHES TO DEVELOPING PROFESSIONAL JUDGEMENT

TECHNICAL RATIONAL PERSPECTIVE VERSUS PROFESSIONAL ARTISTRY

For the midwife, there is real dilemma in trying to formalise the professional judgement process where the midwife is so familiar with both the clinical and objective data as well as being in a close professional relationship with the woman (Kirkham et al. 2002, Mong-Chue 2000). Therefore, for midwives making professional judgements, this not only involves the woman and relevant family members but also the midwives themselves (Axten 2000, Cioffi and Markham 1997, Price and Price 1997). The midwife is in a key position to gather together information from a range of resources, research, existing knowledge and clinical observations, and may add to this a more psychological or intuitive impression. It has been argued that, as the judgement and decision-making becomes more urgent, the approach to the judgement becomes more **rational** and analytical (Buckingham and Adams 2000a, Eraut 1990). In these cases, information from sources other than verifiable evidence may not or cannot always be sought, so that the part of the process that is already the most difficult to identify and explain is also the part most often disregarded.

Nursing and midwifery are often described as containing the values pertaining to both art and science. Within this concept, a useful description is the differentiation between knowing 'how' – something which can be tested or measured as a skill and encompasses the 'art' form of nursing and midwifery and knowing 'that' – where knowledge is grounded in theory and empirical research and supports the scientific elements of nursing or

midwifery practice (McKenna 1997). From the professional viewpoint, this is all related to the experiences and status of the individual and the professional standards against which the judgement would be compared. This is discussed later in the chapter.

As part of the 'art' of practice, there should be significant time on most occasions for the process of making a judgement to take place. Where this is the case, greater emphasis can be placed on the other forms of evidence that might be available for both women and the healthcare professional. This may include the use of reflection in an attempt to understand much deeper processes than might be apparent initially (Lyons 1999, Schon 1983), although the use of reflection (see Chapter 10) has been criticised as being too reliant on intuition and not reliant enough on salient fact and 'real time' knowledge (Price 1995).

REASONING AND CRITICAL THINKING

Alongside unequivocal information – where this exists – there may also be a need to assess the likely effects of taking a certain line of action, based on the risk or probability of certain outcomes occurring. Taken from the cognitive perspective there is an attempt to rationalise the 'pros and cons' of the situation (Beck 1998, Crow et al. 1995). Later in the process, and especially where there is the addition of new information, interpretation of the data will apportion its significance to include, reject or suspend judgement related to its relevance (Thompson 1999). **Reasoning** (internal debate) is another way of making sense of or ordering the information, but it may not always be clear whether the information being debated is accurate or trustworthy and so there is an element of trying to 'second guess' the effect of the intended action on the outcome (Mong-Chue 2000). There is also concern that this approach can involve the opinion of the healthcare professional rather than a display of the information that is unbiased and also accessible and understandable to all those involved in the process. This might include midwives as well as women where highly technical medical or other information is being processed to project the probability of risk. For example, there is the use of presumption – something that might happen, the degree to which it is likely to happen stacked against the events around what has already happened and the research evidence that supports this. When exploring the decision-making process around the practice of episiotomy, Barwise (1998) challenges the responsibility of the individual midwife to be up to date with current research and be accountable for its inclusion or omission from their practice (see Chapter 3). However, as identified by Mander (1995) and discussed by Newton et al. (2000), the majority of midwives can only practice within agreed employment boundaries that are likely to limit their freedom to make decisions that are not in line with employment policy. Future changes in how practice is regulated by the NMC will also have an effect (Opoku 2003, NMC 2004b).

PROFESSIONAL JUDGEMENT IN EDUCATION

From personal experience both as a student and an educator, it has been recognised that education involves a range of judgements and decisions at various levels. These may not relate to a clinical situations *per se*, but they affect those who will, in due course, be making them. One recent development in midwifery education has been the introduction of **problem- or enquiry-based learning (PBL/EBL)**, where clearly identifiable clinical situations are used in order to educate and stimulate enquiry that is based in the classroom setting but relates to the clinical reality (Fraser and Cooper 2003). This is in contrast to the conventional approach where there is a reliance on education based upon learning about care as a task-related entity and where these militate against the development of critical observation and enquiry (Burroughs and Hoffbrand 1990, Cioffi 1998). This is laudable where the profession of midwifery, although highly reliant on a sound knowledge of basic physiology and anatomy, has to apply that to the inconsistent nature of the individual. Education therefore allows the student to learn about a range of likely scenarios that will include the possibilities of rare phenomena as well as the common and normal. It is only where there is an in-depth understanding of all these factors that judgements in the clinical setting can be viewed as reliable and can be depended on by the practitioner (Cioffi and Markham 1997, Cioffi 1998). However, there is a need to make transparent the process that exists from the point where the student is offered, or has access, to the information and then seeing that there is sufficient ability to synthesise and adapt that knowledge in practice. It is at this point that the educator's own knowledge and value systems come into play. This part of the education of students is most important where it continues into the clinical environment where all midwives, regardless of their individual characteristics or abilities, will act as role models to the student through mentorship.

Without a verifiable system to assess student knowledge and skills in a range of formats, this 'judgement' system – of competence in the given field – cannot be verified. Therefore, the attainment of competence needs to be compared with others at the same stage of learning if an agreed standard of acceptable knowledge is to be attained. The student then has to demonstrate the capacity to adapt that knowledge accordingly to reach the professional standard that a midwife needs to make valid and reliable judgements and decisions in the clinical setting.

One criticism of any scoring framework that tries to assess achievement is the use of cognitive values that range, for example: from excellent at the top level to poor at the other end of the scale. Unless these are set against levels of achievement that are agreed and acknowledged by the midwifery profession as a whole, they will produce midwives whose individual professional standards vary. Where midwives work within an agreed framework of best practice upheld within a statutory framework of professional conduct, there is a need for this to be a national standard. The recent introduction of professional competencies has made great strides in this area and has largely been led by educationalists (United Kingdom Central Council for Nursing, Midwifery and Health Visiting [UKCC] 1999). The effect of judgements on the progress and esteem of students should never be underestimated (Davies and Atkinson 1991, Cavanagh and Snape 1997). The process of how students are judged, both academically and clinically, still appears to fall short of being a transparent and enabling process that assesses the skills and competencies as required by the qualified midwife in practice (Anderson 1999). The introduction and success of some mentoring schemes and the use of preceptorship may address this issue, but these are currently linked more to individual institutions than to national consensus. Professional judgement and subsequent decision making in the educational environment must arguably be the most transparent of all as there is ample time to prepare, undertake and assess critical tests that will aid vital judgements and for some students, very final decisions. All of these steps should be open to scrutiny so that the student, at whatever level of education, can develop and move forward as part of the process. Where the decision recommends registration or graduation, the educational experience will be the foundation for that midwife's future. Where the decision is made to fail or remove students from programmes, it must be because it is the individual attributes and competence of the student that have been appropriately measured and found to be inadequate, rather than this being from a failure of them to 'fit into' the system (Cavanagh and Snape 1997, Kelly 1999).

Any judgement should be about whether a student (at any level) has demonstrated skills or knowledge that meet or exceed an already agreed standard, and that the degree to which the student has acquired this knowledge or competence can be measured. Where the knowledge is largely based on fact, fairly right or wrong forms of information, all students can undertake tests that offer them an equal chance of success, as with the use of multiple choice questions and to some degree, with essay-style answers in examination papers. In the more diverse forms of assignments, the assessment is more related to the comprehension of the student about key concepts, and greater analysis of the information than that needed to recall lists of facts and figures. It is at this point that the process of judgement begins to be important, and once the framework errs from what is clearly a right or wrong fact, the assessor has to rely on how near or how far the student is from an accepted level of understanding. Who sets the ranges for this level, maintains and owns them will all contribute to the process of judgement of the student's ability or level of knowledge. Increasingly, education in the fields of the health sciences appears to be more diverse and includes varied ways not only to test their knowledge but also to help them develop skills for lifelong learning and for use in their practice. Where the less formal frameworks are used within the educational establishment, arguably it is even more important to look at how judgements are made about the student's ability and progress. The more open the educational tool, the more it is subject to a process of judgement that may no longer be focused on the ability and knowledge of the student but on how the student has approached or undertaken the task. Although these factors might be important for the student's overall development, the distinction needs to be made between judgement of the student's ability and the student's characteristics. This can be demonstrated very clearly where students are asked to do any form of verbal presentation. In making a judgement about a pass or fail approach, the framework of marking must be explicit – to both the student and the assessor, about the standard that is required. Therefore, if the student is being assessed on appearance, the expected standard of dress must be explained. However, if this has not been included within the assessment standard and has not been clarified as part of the marking criteria, it must not then form part of the judgement process if a student turns up in what the assessor thinks is inappropriate dress and adds this as a value to the assessment.

There is perhaps a need for some retrospection and reflection within the educational fields for the role that professional judgement plays in lifelong learning and professional development. Where assessment criteria are used these need to be clearly identified with measurable goals or competencies so that an overall standard can be identified. Where judgement is given as a concrete value (e.g. 75%, or excellent) these values must be transparent. What has contributed to it being worth that much/little? Where judgement is not applicable as having a discrete value as above, but is more of an overall standard issue, the standard must be explicable. Where the student has met, exceeded or failed to meet it, the components that led to such a judgement must also be demonstrable. Where midwifery education can demonstrate such a framework, the use of reliable and consistent approaches can then be seen as transferable to other areas in clinical practice.

PROFESSIONAL JUDGEMENT IN MANAGEMENT

Judgement in the context of management and midwives is discussed here more in relation to the midwifery manager's wider professional responsibilities. This may also include statutory supervision as a Supervisor of Midwives. The midwife with managerial responsibilities may not have a single professional allegiance but may be required to juggle these according to pressing or required priorities from other domains. Where there is a hierarchical framework, both managerially and medically, the allegiance will be primarily to the employer; this might be from the local Primary Health Care Trust or its equivalent and continuing upwards to the DoH. Alongside this managerial pathway, allegiances will also be made with other colleagues from a range of disciplines, professional and non-professional as well as to the local population (see Chapters 8 and 11).

The process of judgement is likely to be affected by these allegiances, for example, they may exert pressure on an individual's personal circumstances in a direct way where their employment is more reliant on their performance as a manager than on their clinical skills as a midwife. Within the current healthcare environment, some of the guesswork of judgement has been removed by a much closer adherence to policy initiatives and the overt introduction of evidence-based practices and the concept of risk (DoH 1997, 1998, Johanson and Rigby 1999, Symon 1998). Once these concepts are introduced into the equation, the judgement process becomes considerably more in line with the **hypothetico-deductive model.** This might not necessarily be the way that midwives would want to undertake judgement about the provision of care services, but this quite rigid and formal structure is now in place and forms part of what is now conventional care management (Greenhalgh 2002). Managers may also have to reconcile competing priorities between different services when deciding how to allocate resources. In this respect, the decisions – however well considered – may not always be popular.

Professional discipline also requires professional leadership, and this may involve the judgement of an individual professional's conduct when viewed as having fallen below the agreed standard of the midwifery profession. The midwife in management has a responsibility to contribute to the overall function of the professional body for midwifery practice by being the gate-keeper of these standards and taking action where this is required. This may involve referral to the NMC where cases of misconduct will be judged by a Professional Conduct Committee, the ultimate judgement being to remove the professional from practice (Bolam v. Friern Hospital Management Committee 1957, Effken 2001, Pyne 1992). In judging professionals for their conduct, Pyne (1992: 11) noted that assessing misconduct was a challenge in ". . . a profession whose practitioners must be constantly engaged in the exercise of personal judgement, and in an often imperfect environment."

This raises the conflict between professional and personal values and the role of each with regard to the acts of the professional in practice.

It also highlights the crucial determination by the statutory body of what constitutes autonomy: for the profession and for the professional (see Chapter 1). Midwives have clear delineations for what is accepted as appropriate activities of the midwife and sphere of practice (NMC 2004a, NMC 2004b). Although these are clearly defined on paper, such clarity is not so apparent in practice where the organisation of care is in conflict with the approach to and context of care that could be provided by midwives (Homer and Davis 1999).

PROFESSIONAL JUDGEMENT IN CLINICAL PRACTICE

Once the agreed standards for registration have been met, the newly qualified midwife is seen as competent to make professional judgements (NMC 2004b). The recognition of a probationary period is professional acknowledgement that judgement is a skill in its own right that will need to be developed over time. It is to be hoped that the probationary midwife will have a foundation of experiences and reflections upon which to base a new career. The ethos of life long learning is that this will be an on-going process occurring at differing levels in relation to the individual and the midwifery role. The expectation is that the initial foundation of knowledge will be used as a base upon which to build what will become the core for midwifery skill and expertise (Steele 1997).

Alongside the midwife's professional identity there is also each individual's experiences, attitudes and insights. It would be naïve not to consider the effects of these on the professional judgement process (Kirkham et al. 2002). Another consideration is the relationship to those the midwife is caring for in a professional role, and the degree of authority or control in this. With the advocacy of informed choice for all women within the maternity services, for midwives there is a very well-formed debate about this, as noted previously. Although this may be explicit for the profession,

it might not always fit so comfortably with individual practitioners (Levy 1999). The increased involvement of women in their own healthcare where the 'system' has historically been largely patriarchal, means that it is now accepted and advocated that judgements related to a woman's choice cannot be made by the professional (DoH 1993, House of Commons 2003, DoH 2004, NMC 2004b). Therefore, although the woman's choice may be inexplicable to the health professional and not in line with their professional advice and knowledge, they have to respect that this is the woman's choice and that the decision about that choice rests with her (see Chapter 9).

The process of making judgements and ultimately decisions varies according to the degree of the individual's involvement (will it affect you, or are you just a bystander?) and the level of responsibility that you have regarding your professional or social status (what have you to lose – your credibility, your professional registration, your job or possibly all three?).

In the process of professional judgement, the ability to make a judgement does not follow quite the same line as some of the models suggested for the process itself. The ability probably could also be described as the way all the information is assessed according to its importance and relevance to further action. Sometimes, it is possible to make a judgement but not to reach a decision as a result of that judgement. See the following example in Box 6.1.

Where knowledge is limited, it may be easy to make a judgement: to summarise what information you do have and finally come to a conclusion. Consider, for example, an extensive antepartum haemorrhage (APH). The judgement about the clinical condition would be immediate, and it would not be appropriate to seek out more information than the essential before making the decision that would initiate action. In less acute circumstances there is more time to gather together the range of information that will inform your judgement and lead to your decision. Where this is the case, it is whether you know the extent or deficit of

Box 6.1

Sunita visits the antenatal clinic and has recently arrived from Bangladesh. From a very brief initial conversation you make the judgement that she speaks very little English. At that point, *you do not instigate any tests/investigations because informed consent could not be obtained.* Later, because you will need to be able to communicate with her, you will use that judgement to decide what to do about it, such as involving an interpreter.

your knowledge – whether you might be aware that there is something you do not know and can take this into account that will affect your *ability* to make the judgement. It is at this point that the decision might be to refer to someone with greater knowledge.

The current philosophy that underpins the National Health Service (NHS) is based around the issues of clinical governance and research evidence (DoH 1997, 1998). Whenever a person enters into the remit of NHS care, there is now an onus of responsibility from the most senior level of Government to the newly qualified professional that this care will involve the use of research as evidence when making professional judgements (see Chapter 3). Research studies have evaluated interventions, explored associations between disease and social factors and described effects of care with regard to physical and psychological outcomes. The degree to which the findings have been disseminated into the environment where care is taking place, affects to some extent how that knowledge will be used as part of the judgement process and whether professionals judge it as being useful and effective in the clinical setting (Appleton and Cowley 2003). There are now many examples of what is seen to be the highest or 'gold' standards, from undertaking quantitative studies using randomised controlled trails (RCTs) to qualitative research such as observation studies. These feed into the pool of knowledge and are in some instances adopted as part of professional,

and often Government policy such as **National Institute of Clinical Excellence** (NICE) guidelines. At this point, judgements about *what* evidence to use is taken away from the individual or professional group (Symon 1998). An example of this would be the use of steroids where there is a risk of pre-term labour. To assist in making a decision towards such a case, decision trees have been created (see Chapter 5). These are in the form of a flow chart of care that assist in directing the health professional towards appropriate care, as well as being a transparent report of the care given and decisions made along the way (Bonner 2001, Thompson 1999, Torrance and Dockery 2003). However, in order to follow the decision tree, or similar protocols or guidelines, the judgement is then not about the decision to treat but about whether the woman is actually at risk of the condition itself. In the case of pre-term labour and the use of steroids, the diagnosis of pre-term labour relies on the skilled health professional alongside the experiences of the woman to verify the actual clinical situation. This might not be straightforward; the observations might be difficult to interpret and the attending professionals may have differing degrees of skills and expectations with regard to their role and status.

Exploring this pre-term labour scenario further, should the woman also be obese there can be difficulty establishing the frequency of contractions. Furthermore, if the woman is also experiencing vaginal bleeding with the potential risk of an APH, this might preclude performing a vaginal examination to assess the state of the cervix, except with a speculum (which may not give the best information). These are examples of the grey areas where it is the health professionals' skills that are important as part of the process of making the judgement, however, they may not be sufficient. What does the midwife do? This is the process of judgement and decision. At each point the midwife weighs up the evidence before them to make a probabilistic assessment (see Chapter 5) for or against the probability of the symptom indicating pre-term labour. Taking each single piece of evidence into account should help to create the whole picture that will inform the judgement process and indicate the direction for action. Where pre-term labour is a strong probability, the decision is then clear and treatment must be given as denoted by Trust or other policy. Where it is subsequently identified that an error in judgement was made, strategies need to be in place to review all the evidence available at that time in order to identify whether there was any fault in the process as a whole. For this a record of the evidence and decision making process by those who made the judgement would be needed (NMC 2004c). This is sometimes pre-empted in current clinical settings where there is a critical incident risk report required by the Trust in accordance with the **Clinical Negligence Scheme for Trusts (CNST)** (DoH 1996). This approach aims to be pro-active by acknowledging that the process of judgement might not have been straightforward, as previously noted by Pyne (1992) and the emphasis is to replace what has been viewed as a culture more inclined to blame, to one that provides understanding and support (Fyle et al. 2002).

Alongside research evidence are the midwife's own personal past experiences and observations. These should be drawn upon when needed, with some editing in the form of critical reflection or review (Lyons 1999). Experiences are not so useful at a later stage unless they have been evaluated with regard to the outcome and how this relates to the current enquiry. Memories are not the same as professional experience where the professional will have built on the experience, they will have sought to understand why and how it happened and to have made mental notes of the positive and negative outcomes from it. Memories could be considered more as nostalgic monographs that are too often one-dimensional where they focus on the self rather than the situation. Making a clear distinction between memories and experience, the professional will develop and apply their knowledge when needed, rather than displaying all their

Box 6.2

Sally has requested an epidural for pain relief in labour, and asks you for information before the procedure. You expect that most women would have had information about this prior to their labour, but as this is not apparent in Sally's case, you proceed to give her information as to the procedure, its risks and benefits.

You remember a recent shift on labour ward where you witnessed a woman experience a reaction to epidural analgesia in the form of severe hypotension.

• Do you inform Sally of this potential risk as she appears to be more distressed with her labour?

knowledge regardless of need, as in the example in Box 6.2.

In this situation, even though the midwife has a responsibility to inform Sally of any potential risks, it would not be appropriate for her to give an account of the hypotensive episode in detail at the point Sally was about to need an epidural. A judgement needs to be made about the degree and depth of information Sally needs and then the decision to inform her to this level, with the knowledge that potentially a serious effect could occur.

Consider the following examples from clinical practice in terms of how the midwife might exercise professional judgement. They are offered as points for discussion or personal refection with regard to the likely process of making a judgement and the subsequent course of events.

CASE SCENARIOS FROM PRACTICE

Case Scenario 6.1

You are working on night duty on the labour ward. At about 11 pm you answer the phone and Jane speaks to you.

'Hello, I am worried, I am 23 weeks pregnant and I cannot feel the baby moving, do you think it is alright?'

- What action do you take?
- What other information do you need to know?
- What research evidence is there in relation to fetal movement: is this relevant at 23 weeks' gestation?
- Is there a policy about reduced fetal movements? Is it appropriate in Jane's case?
- What is your professional judgement?
- Where will you record all the information obtained in this situation?

In this situation there is the difficulty of not actually being able to see Jane, and so any information obtained is already limited. In reaching a judgement, what other information do you need to know and what background knowledge or research evidence could you use to assess the situation? For fetal movement studies, there is quite a body of knowledge, but how relevant is this at 23 weeks' gestation? You also need to be aware of any policy about reduced fetal movements and your own sphere of practice in this situation. With regard to the initial contact being a telephone call, involving you making a professional judgment, where will you record all this information?

In the following Scenario 6.2, one word is different in each version of the otherwise similar request. Consider what effect (if any) the difference might make to the outcome.

Case Scenario 6.2   Non-Clinical Judgement

You are the named midwife for Kate and her baby girl, Isobel on a busy postnatal ward. At 10:30 am the access bell rings, although visiting time is not until 6 pm. However, husbands/partners may visit throughout the day.

- What do you think you may do if faced with the following requests?

"Hello: I know it isn't visiting time, but my sister Kate has just had her baby and I have to go back to Delhi tonight, could I see her for a few minutes?"

"Hello: I know it isn't visiting time, but my sister Kate has just had her baby and I have to go back to Sweden tonight, could I see her for a few minutes?"

"Hello: I know it isn't visiting time, but my sister Kate has just had her baby and I have to go back to New York tonight, could I see her for a few minutes?"

"Hello: I know it isn't visiting time, but my sister Kate has just had her baby and I have to go back to look after my own children, could I see her for just a few minutes?"

- Think through how you may respond given each request.
- Consider what response(s) another midwife may make when also faced with these requests.

When making non-clinical judgements, the response given may reflect your position within the environment, your own self-esteem, and how you perceive your role as an empathetic supportive advocate to the woman. However, if you make the judgement that the visit has a valid claim and you decide to let the visitor in, your decision may be based on certain conditions – that is, that you go with the visitor to see Kate, you may need to ask other women if they mind a visitor entering the room they share with Kate, or you may ask Kate to receive her visitor in an alternative room. You may also need to explain your action/decision to other staff in the area. Finally, reflect on the possible differences that the information given by the visitor in each situation could have on the judgement and ultimate decision you made. You may also wish to reflect on the appropriateness of the 6 pm visiting policy.

Case Scenario 6.3

You have just come back on duty on a busy antenatal/post-natal ward following 2 weeks annual leave, and as a result do not know any of the women on the ward.

As you prepare to take report from the morning shift, a healthcare assistant calls from the corridor:

'The woman in room 10, she is haemorrhaging!"

You look around but cannot see any of your colleagues in the vicinity.

What will you do?

It is usual to gather together what knowledge you have; this might be in the form of written records that will give you information about past events and current physical status, such as the woman's haemoglobin level or the position of the fetus or the placenta. You also have a choice of physical observations that will add to your understanding of the current situation – these might be relevant maternal observations, a key one being the amount and appearance of the blood, and a pulse rate. In an antenatal situation you might want to undertake some form of fetal monitoring and ensure that the woman is in the best position to reduce the effects on the fetus. Until someone else comes to your aid (and will they if you have not directed the healthcare assistant to do this?), identify what you would utilise to assist your judgement of the situation when you first make contact with the woman.

CONCLUSION

Throughout this chapter, reference has been made to a number of models, largely used in nursing, that incorporate a philosophical approach to the theory of judgement and decision making. To be useful in practice, these theories need to be made applicable to the clinical situation so that the health professional can feel more reassured that they are making a professional judgement and not one that has arisen by luck or chance, or one that has been imposed upon them (Woodhall 1999). The professional judgement will follow a defined process that can be called upon, if needed, to support their action and that can be reviewed in retrospect. Regardless of the source of knowledge, or in fact its reliability, the process of accumulating facts upon which a judgement will be made, regarding the needs of the health professional, follows a fairly simple process. However this process may have been defined, it relies on the collection of information and its distillation for analysis and relevance in order to reach resolution at that point in time.

With regard to the scenarios presented, where the process that led to the judgement and subsequent decision and action can be tracked and substantiated, the professionalism of the individual can also be demonstrated. Furthermore, where the actions can be compared to those taken by another person with similar qualifications and experience this continues to form the view that the judgement made was valid. There might be errors in the interpretation or weighting of the information available, or information that should have been taken into account might not have been, but where even a basic record of the process is available, this forms the ethos of the Bolam standard expected of the professional in the clinical situation against the expert 'from the outside'.

It follows that where there is clear line of accountability for the judgement, this should lead to transparency in what was decided about the action. Where there is a mis-match, this might be because of a lack of skill to convert the judgement into action. Where the record is unclear or absent it is possible that such events can still be explained and understood, however, it is the responsibility of the accountable professional to ensure that this occurs.

KEY POINTS FOR BEST PRACTICE

- In the professional context, judgement is part of a process that involves the critical analysis of information and the potential outcome in order to come to a decision.

- This process may be ordered and lengthy or almost instantaneous, based on the clinical setting.

- The autonomy of women and their families, as recipients of care, should be acknowledged within the judgement-making process.

- The individual health professional (whether in education, management or clinical practice) may be constrained in this process by outside influences that relate to policy, procedure or professional standards.

- The competence and expertise of the health professional is likely to have an effect on their ability to make judgements and take decisions.

- Accurate and contemporaneous documentation of the decision process is essential.

- Assessment as to whether a judgement or decision was right is probably only possible in retrospect, when the individual circumstances are taken into account.

- Undertaking reflective practice can assist on-going professional development and expertise in making clinical judgements.

References

Anderson T 1999 Are we training competent midwives? The Practising Midwife 2(10): 4–5.

Appleton J, Cowley S 2003 Valuing professional judgement in health visiting practice. Community Practitioner 76(6): 215–220.

Axten S 2000 The thinking midwife: arriving at judgement. British Journal of Midwifery 8(5): 287–290.

Barker W 2001 Measurement or intuition? Community Practitioner 74(8): 291–293.

Barwise C 1998 Episiotomy and decision making. British Journal of Midwifery 6(12): 787–790.

Beck C 1998 Intuition in nursing practice: sharing graduate student exemplars with undergraduate student. Journal of Nurse Education 37(4): 169–173.

Benner P 1982 From novice to expert. American Journal of Nursing 82: 402–407.

Benner P, Tanner C 1987 Clinical judgement: how expert nurses use intuition. American Journal of Nursing 87(1): 23–31.

Bolam v. Friern Hospital Management Committee 1957 2 All England Law Report 118.

Bolitho v. City and Hackney Health Authority 1997 3 Weekly Law Report 1151.

Bonner G 2001 Decision making for health care professionals: use of decision trees within the community mental health setting. Journal of Advanced Nursing 35(3): 349–356.

Buckingham C, Adams A 2000a Classifying clinical decision making: a unifying approach. Journal of Advanced Nursing 32(4): 981–989.

Buckingham C, Adams A 2000b Classifying clinical decision making: interpreting nursing intuition, heuristics and medical diagnosis. Journal of Advanced Nursing 32(4): 990–998.

Burroughs J, Hoffbrand BI 1990 A critical look at nursing observations. Postgraduate Medical Journal 66: 370–372.

Cavanagh S, Snape J 1997 Educational sources of stress in midwifery students. Nurse Education Today 17(2): 128–134.

Celador International. 2003 39 Long Acre, London, WC2E 9LG, www.celador.co.uk.

Charles C, Gafni A, Whelan T 1997 Shared-decision making in the medical encounter: What does it mean? Social Science and Medicine 44(5): 681–692.

Cioffi J 1998 Education for clinical decision making in midwifery practice. Midwifery 14(1): 18–22.

Cioffi J, Markham R 1997 Clinical decision-making by midwives: managing case complexity. Journal of Advanced Nursing 25(2): 265–272.

Crow R, Chase J, Lamond D 1995 The cognitive component of nursing assessment: an analysis. Journal of Advanced Nursing 22(2): 206–212.

Davies RM, Atkinson P 1991 Students of midwifery: doing the obs and other coping strategies. Midwifery 7(3): 113–121.

Dimond B 2001 Who is setting the standard for maternity care? British Journal of Midwifery 9(4): 245–248.

Department of Health 1993 Changing Childbirth – a report

of the expert maternity group. HMSO, London.

Department of Health Statutory Instrument 1996 No. 251 The National Health Service (Clinical Negligence Scheme) Regulations 1996.

Department of Health 1997 The New NHS. Modern, Dependable. HMSO, London.

Department of Health 1998 A First Class Service – Quality in the new NHS. HMSO, London.

Department of Health 2004 National Service Framework for Children, Young People and Maternity Services: executive summary. DoH, London.

Effken L 2001 Informational basis for expert intuition. Journal of Advanced Nursing 34(2): 246–255.

Eraut M 1990 Identifying the knowledge which underpins performance. In: Black H (ed), Knowledge and competencies: Current issues in training and education. HMSO, London, pp. 22–28.

Fraser D, Cooper M 2003 The Midwife. In: Fraser D, Cooper M (eds), Myles Textbook for Midwives, 14th edition. Churchill Livingstone, Edinburgh, pp. 3–11.

Friend J 1995 Respect for women's choice. Maternal and Child Health 20(6): 202–204, 206.

Fyle J, McGlynn AG, Jokinen M 2002 Flying lessons: risk management and the NPSA. RCM Midwives 5(10): 322–323.

Gillon R 1994 Medical ethics: four principles plus attention to scope. British Medical Journal 309: 184–188.

Greenhalgh T 2002 Intuition and evidence – uneasy bedfellows. British Journal of General Practice 52(478): 395–400.

Harding D 2000 Making choices in childbirth. In: Page L (ed), The New Midwifery – Science and Sensitivity in Practice. Churchill Livingstone, Edinburgh, pp. 71–85.

Homer C, Davis G 1999 Can elective labour induction be woman-centred? British Journal of Midwifery 7(11): 686–689.

House of Commons Health Committee 2003 Choice in Maternity Services: Ninth Report. The Stationery Office, London.

Johanson R, Rigby C 1999 Clinical governance in practice: achieving sustainable quality in maternity. Journal of Clinical Excellence 1(1): 19–22.

Kelly AV 1999 The Curriculum, Theory and Practice. Assessment Evaluation, Appraisal and Accountability. 4th edition. London: Sage, pp. 28–164.

King L, Appleton J 1997 Intuition: a critical review of the research and rhetoric. Journal of Advanced Nursing 26: 198–202.

Kirkham M, Stapleton H, Curtis P, et al. 2002 Stereotyping as a professional defence mechanism. British Journal of Midwifery 10(9): 549–552.

Kitzinger S 1993 Ourselves as Mothers. The Universal Experience of Motherhood. Bantam Books: London, pp. 1–16.

Levy V 1999 Protective steering: a grounded theory study of the processes by which midwives facilitate informed choices during pregnancy. Journal of Advanced Nursing 29: 104–112

Lyons J 1999 Reflective education for professional practice: discovering knowledge from experience. Nurse Education Today 19(1): 29–34

Mander R 1995 Where does the buck stop? Accountability in midwifery. In: Watson R (ed), Accountability in Nursing Practice. Chapman & Hall, London, pp. 95–106.

McKenna H 1997 Nursing Theories and Models. Routledge, London.

Mong-Chue C 2000 The challenges of midwifery practice for critical thinking. British Journal of Midwifery 8(3): 179–183.

Newton C, Johnson C, Drury C 2000 Responsibilities and accountability. In: Fraser D (ed), Professional Studies in Midwifery practice. Churchill Livingstone, Edinburgh, pp. 95–109.

Nursing and Midwifery Council 2004a Code of Professional Conduct: standards for conduct, performance and ethics. NMC, London.

Nursing and Midwifery Council 2004b Midwives Rules and Standards. NMC, London.

Nursing and Midwifery Council 2004c Guidelines for Records and Record keeping. NMC, London.

Opoku D 2003 The history and regulation of midwifery. In: Fraser D, Cooper M (eds), Myles Textbook for Midwives, 14th edition. Churchill Livingstone, Edinburgh, pp. 77–96.

Page L 2003 Women-centred, midwife-friendly care: principles, patterns and culture of practice. In: Fraser D, Cooper M (eds), Myles Textbook for Midwives, 14th edition. Churchill Livingstone, Edinburgh, pp. 31–48.

Price A 1995 Making midwifery decisions, sound choices. Modern Midwife 10(5): 14–18.

Price A, Price B 1997 Making midwifery decisions. Modern Midwife 7(10): 15–19.

Pyne RH 1992 Professional Discipline in Nursing, Midwifery and Health Visiting. 2nd edition. Blackwell Science, London.

Schon DA 1983 The Reflective Practitioner: how professionals think in action. Basic Books, New York.

Steele R 1997 Continuing professional development – new jargon or a workable reality? RCM Midwives 110: 1314–1317.

Symon A 1998 The role of unit protocols and policies. British Journal of Midwifery 6(10): 631–634.

Symon A 1999 Debate about the current system. British Journal of Midwifery 7(1): 52–56.

Thompson C 1999 A conceptual treadmill: the need for 'middle ground' in clinical decision making theory in nursing. Journal of Advanced Nursing 30(5): 1222–1229.

Thompson C 2001 Clinical decision making in nursing: theoretical perspectives and their relevance to practice – a response to Jean

Harbison. Journal of Advanced Nursing 35(1): 134–137.

Thompson C, McCaughhan D, Cullum N 2001 Research information in nurses' clinical decision-making: what is useful? Journal of Advanced Nursing 36(3): 376–388.

Tingle JH 2002 Do guidelines have legal implications? Archives of Diseases in Childhood 86: 387–388.

Torrance E, Dockery K 2003 Clinical governance and caesarean section. British Journal of Midwifery 11(2): 94–96.

Trede F, Higgs J 2003 Re-framing the clinician's role in collaborative clinical decision making: re-thinking practice knowledge and the notion of clinician-patient relationships. Learning in Health and Social Care 2(2): 66–73.

Vandenbussche F, Jong-Potjer L, Stiggelbout A, et al. 1999 Differences in the valuation of birth outcomes among pregnant women, mothers and obstetricians. Birth 26(3): 178–183.

Van de Vusse L 1999 Decision making in analyses of women's birth stories. Birth 26(1): 43–50.

Woodhall T 1999 Who should decide? Decision making in the event of unexpected stillbirth: a reflective exercise. Journal of Neonatal Nursing 5(4): 18–22.

United Kingdom Central Council for Nursing, Midwifery and Health Visiting 1999 Fitness for Practice UKCC Commission for Nursing and Midwifery Education. UKCC, London.

Further Reading

Opoku D 2003 The history and regulation of midwifery. In: Fraser D, Cooper M. (eds), Myles Textbook for Midwives, 14th edition. Churchill Livingstone, Edinburgh. pp. 77–96.

This chapter not only describes the past but also makes challenging observations about the future and the changes that will occur as the Nursing and Midwifery Council becomes fully effective. It is a useful source for midwives to consider how these changes might affect the evaluation of their professional judgement and decision making as well as the standard of clinical competence expected.

Barwise C 1998 Episiotomy and decision making. British Journal of Midwifery 6(12): 787– 790.

Although the procedure of undertaking an episiotomy is now relatively uncommon, not so long ago it was considered appropriate and was performed routinely by midwives in some instances. This paper is included for the approach used to explore decision making in a practical setting and how the midwife contributed to such changes in practice.

Midwives Information and Resource Service 2003 Informed Choice Initiative. Bristol, MIDIRS (www.MIDIRS.org).

This is a revision of the original Informed Choice leaflets now consisting of 15 leaflets for health professionals and women with supporting professional development tools for midwives. With regard to professional judgement and decision making, the evidence base for the leaflets aims to equip healthcare professionals with the best available information in order to assist women and their partners to make choices about their care.

Chapter 7

Making Ethical Decisions

Shirley R. Jones

INTRODUCTION

The whole of this book is devoted to various aspects of decision making. It considers different settings and approaches, underlying knowledge, autonomous or partnership decisions and the development of professional judgement and reflection. The aim of this chapter is to concentrate on ensuring that the decisions, made by midwives, in any of these areas have an ethical basis.

WHAT IS AN ETHICAL DECISION?

The premise in this chapter is that any decision is the final point of choice, a precise moment in a period of deliberating on any available options. Therefore, during the deliberations about practicalities, previous experiences, preferences, resources and other factors, there should be room for consideration of ethics. In order to do this, however, it is necessary to have an understanding of what is meant by ethics and morality.

"Ethics is the application of the processes and theories of moral philosophy to a real situation.

It is concerned with the basic principles and concepts that guide human beings in thought and action, and which underlie their **values.**" (Jones 2000: 8).

This definition serves to state the academic position of ethics, leaving us to presume that morality is fundamentally related to matters of conscience. In a theoretical context, this position is acceptable; however, in everyday living and in practice settings there is little evidence of a distinction between morals and ethics. Indeed, as stated by Loughlin (2002), it would be unusual for someone to provide an example of an act that was considered immoral and ethical, or moral yet unethical. Therefore, this chapter will follow the common usage rule of the terms being interchangeable.

It follows then that an ethical decision is one that is underpinned by a moral code or an ethical framework or theory; where consideration has been given to the rights and wrongs of the decision. What constitutes right and wrong, however, is determined by the ethical stance or basic **values** and beliefs of those who are judging that decision. Where midwifery care is concerned, decisions could be judged by the midwife herself, by the woman and her family and relevant members of the healthcare team. There is the potential for a variety of judgements. Such a situation was evident in the high-profile case of conjoined twins, known as Mary and Jodie (Re A (minors) (conjoined twins: separation) [2000]), where decisions being made by doctors, lawyers and judges were open to public scrutiny and met with a wide variety of views. Initially, midwives would have been involved in decisions being made about care and treatment of the mother and then the babies. Where some might have had no difficulty in deciding what they felt was right or wrong, others would have encountered conflicts and **dilemmas**.

CONFLICT IN DECISION MAKING

The case of Mary and Jodie was exceptional; rarely are midwives faced with such extreme **dilemmas**. However, they could be faced with conflict in decision making on a daily basis. Conflict can arise between midwives and the women for whom they are caring, based on their different **values** and beliefs, throughout the continuum of childbearing care. This statement does not mean that there are many antagonistic relationships between women and their midwives, as conflict is usually resolved with discussion and ethical reasoning. It is part of the midwife's role to support women, aware of their own **values** and beliefs but not allowing them to interfere with their care and advice.

✎ Activity 7.1

List all the areas of potential conflict that could be encountered between a midwife and a woman, from the very first meeting to the end of the post-natal period.

It is probable that many entries on your list relate to informed choice in some form. One example of early conflict that you might have listed, could be where a woman requests a mode of birth that is thought to be high risk in view of her history. For instance, a woman with diabetes mellitus may request a home birth; or a woman who has had one vaginal birth with a post-partum haemorrhage (PPH) of 2000 ml, followed by a Caesarean section for failure to progress with a baby weighing 4 kg, might request a water birth. Another example could relate to the various antenatal screening tests. The midwife should be giving factual information, removing bias as much as possible, but she might believe that all women should have all the tests available. When she encounters a woman who does not want any or some of the tests, there may be conflict that must be overcome.

Antenatal screening for human immune deficiency virus (HIV) can create other potential conflict for midwives with their employers. Trusts have national targets to meet, and therefore the Chief Executive Officers (CEO) will expect the tiers of management to cascade the need to meet targets to those with responsibility for counselling the women and ensuring the blood samples are taken. If the midwives counsel the women according to ethical practice, they will ensure that the women make informed choices. In which case, it is probable that a percentage of women will refuse the test, perhaps resulting in Government targets not being met. The conflict, therefore, relates to whether the midwife should continue with appropriate counselling and fail to meet the targets, or whether she should tailor the encounter with the woman to ensure that targets are met.

✎ Activity 7.2

List any other Trust-based conflicts, which would probably include certain policies, e.g. reducing inequalities and targeting deprived areas.

The third general area for everyday conflicts of views relates to other healthcare professionals with whom midwives interact. As midwives work very closely with doctors – particularly obstetricians and paediatricians – this group of professionals is likely to feature at the top of any list you write for this area of conflict, perhaps alongside other midwives.

THE MIDWIFE'S RESPONSIBILITY IN MAKING ETHICAL DECISIONS

Having stated that conflicts are based on differing **values** and beliefs, it is important to state that these **values** and beliefs are not just related to culture, religion and other forms of general socialisation. There are also **values** and beliefs developed with regard to the area in which one works. For instance, a CEO of a Trust may not have quite the same focus as healthcare workers who are in daily contact with the patients and clients of the Trust. The CEO must have a more strategic overview of the effective use of valuable resources and prioritisation of services.

Additionally, there are the different **values** and beliefs between the various healthcare professions. Midwives frequently complain that maternity services should not be based on the medical model of care, as that model is illness-focused and midwifery should be health-focused, while recognising deviations as they occur. In such situations of conflict midwives cannot ignore the problem and leave it unresolved. They have a responsibility to act in accordance with civil law requirements related to the **duty of care**, consent and client confidentiality, which are underpinned by ethics. They also have a responsibility to act in accordance with the Nursing and Midwifery Council's (NMC) rules, codes and guidance, which also have an ethical basis.

HOW CAN MIDWIVES MAKE ETHICAL DECISIONS?

Many midwives may feel that they make ethical decisions on a daily basis, just by use of their own conscience. That is a good place to start and, in urgent situations, it can be a useful tool. However, unless some conscious thought about ethical approaches has been undertaken, an individual's conscience may lead them to do what suits them, rather than what suits the woman. Also, there is the risk of inconsistency of decision making when left to raw conscience alone. According to Velasquez and Andre (2003a: 1), consistency is 'the absence of contradiction'. This point is not suggesting that there is no room for flexibility; on the contrary, using a framework or theory should allow for the individuality of the situation, while reducing the risk of discrimination, inequality and confusion. If a consistent approach is required, then *ad hoc* reasoning or use of conscience or intuition alone is insufficient. Even rules of thumb, called heuristics by Cioffi and Markham (1997), and stated by them to work most of the time, are insufficient as this term is not precise enough. It could be just for 51% of the time, meaning that for 49% of the time it does not work. Midwives need to develop their understanding of ethical approaches to decision making in order to be more certain of achieving ethical practice.

APPROACHES TO ETHICAL DECISION MAKING

There are various approaches to ethics, and there are many basic principles that underpin them all, albeit that the observance of the basic principles differs between and within the different approaches. Four approaches that will be briefly considered here relate to: **principlism**, virtue, duty, and consequentialism.

THE PRINCIPLES APPROACH (PRINCIPLISM)

In this approach, of the many principles available, four have been selected as being fundamental. Where difficulties with any one of the principles is encountered, consideration of how they impinge on each other in the specific circumstances assists the resolution of conflict.

(i) Autonomy

Autonomy, or respect for it, acknowledges that most people can determine their own needs and goals and that, at least in democratic societies, they are self-governed and **rational**. Respect for autonomy requires that people should not be used as a means to someone else's ends (Jones 2000), but that they should be supported to make decisions that enable them to meet their own needs. This principle is a relative newcomer to the health service, which has been notoriously **paternalistic** (i.e. purporting to know what is best for everyone). The observance of this principle establishes the obligations related to information giving, consent, privacy and confidentiality (Beauchamp and Childress 2001).

(ii) Beneficence

Beneficence has always been one of two underlying principles of the healthcare system. It appears to be a sound principle for midwifery practice, providing an obligation that all actions are for the good of the person or people involved. Conflict could arise, of course, when the required action carries an element of risk or cost to the woman or the baby. For instance, in cases where women require answers to questions that can only be gained by invasive diagnostic tests, each of which carries a percentage risk of miscarriage. Another example could be the administration of pethidine in labour, as the method of pain relief chosen by the woman. Following the administration there could be side effects for the mother and the fetus/neonate, possibly continuing a negative effect into the neonatal period and creating difficulty for the woman who wanted to breastfeed. However, where the woman makes an informed, autonomous choice, the actions may still be beneficent. Further conflict is possible when doing something beneficent for one person causes harm to another.

(iii) Non-maleficence

Non-maleficence calls upon midwives to do no harm, and is the other fundamental principle of the healthcare system, referred to above. In midwifery it is a principle that we would expect to uphold. One of the problems with this principle, especially in conjunction with beneficence, is that the midwife's view of what is doing good and avoiding harm may not match with the views of some of the women for whom they provide care. Screening is an example of this conflict within and between principles. Midwives, and other healthcare professionals, might believe that finding out the ratio of risk of certain abnormalities, with the potential for termination of an abnormal fetus if that is the woman's choice, is both beneficent and non-maleficent. Some women, however, who feel that anxiety levels have been raised unnecessarily, or where a false sense of security has been created, might feel that they were led into a sequence of events that were, for them, harmful (maleficent). In addition, many investigations and treatments have possible side effects that could be harmful; it is essential, therefore, to consider the balance of costs and benefits when making decisions. It is also essential that adequate information regarding risks and benefits is given to women to enable them to make choices from the outset.

(iv) Justice

Justice is a principle that includes fair play of all kinds. Prevention of negative discrimination and creation of equality are the intentions. However, there are different ways of considering what constitutes equality. It depends on the goal to be achieved. For instance, if the goal of equality in antenatal preparation is to achieve equal provision of care and information to all women who attend for care, then we must provide the same amount of everything to everyone. If, on the other hand, the goal is to get all the women to the same level of knowledge and understanding, so that they can all make truly informed choices for and during labour, then the provision must be unequal. In this second example, the women who are pro-active, perhaps better educated and with access to more information sources, would require less provision than those women who are at the other end of the scales. Arguably, both approaches could be deemed right, according to the goal to be achieved.

Some commentators disapprove of **principlism**, stating that it creates a rigid approach by a 'slavish worship of rules' (Velasquez and Andre 2003b: 1), though others feel that principles are too open to interpretation and not directive enough (Clouser and Gert 1994). Hanford (1993) also believes that **principlism** fails to promote and enhance a caring environment. However, for the novice in ethical thinking, it can be a useful place to start until further development can be achieved. It certainly provides a basis for a midwife to justify her decisions and actions.

THE VIRTUE APPROACH

This approach, based on the views of Aristotle, relies on attitudes and character that develop with experience of life, both personal and professional. Examples of virtues are: "... honesty, courage, compassion, generosity, fidelity, integrity, fairness, self-control and prudence."

(Velasquez and Andre 2003b: 1). These virtues should then be applied to decisions and actions with the common good in mind. According to Beauchamp and Childress (2001), an action is only truly virtuous if the motive of the person is proper. They state that someone who performs a morally good act because they know they should, while possibly disliking being in the position of needing to do it, rather than through a deeply held belief that it is the right action, is morally correct but not virtuous.

It is possible that many midwives already function according to virtues; the existence of these virtues being what attracted them to a healthcare profession in the first place. However, it is not a certainty that every midwife has all the necessary virtues. This is not the approach for someone who wants a direct answer to 'what should I do?', as it could be seen as similar to using conscience alone.

THE DUTY-BASED APPROACH

Commonly used in biomedical ethics, **deontology** has a number of strands, from adherence to one supreme principle (**rational** monism), as in Kantianism where autonomy is paramount, to observance of a number of principles that have become duties (pluralism). Pluralist approaches include observance of religious codes as well as the model by Ross (1930), that includes seven *prima facie* equal duties that can be prioritised according to the circumstances and the intuition of the individual, should conflict of duties occur.

In this approach, the duty to the individual is the priority – there is no room for consideration of others who might be affected by the decisions or actions. The intention of the action is what is judged, not the consequences. For instance, if it is felt that one has a duty to tell the truth, then it should be done; the fact that the consequence of telling the truth might be that harm is caused, is not a factor for consideration. However, in Ross's model (1930), as there is room for case-based reasoning (casuistry) and prioritisation of the *prima facie* duties, it inevitably gives the opportunity to avoid the harm that could be caused by slavish worship of duties.

It could be suggested that, even without the underlying knowledge of **deontology**, many midwives have a natural tendency towards this theory. Clinical midwives, in particular, being aware of their **duty of care** for the mothers and babies with whom they have a professional relationship, observe the general duties that protagonists of this theory support. These duties are part of the overall **duty of care** and can be discerned in the Code of Professional conduct: Standards for Conduct, Performance and Ethics (NMC 2004a).

THE CONSEQUENTIAL APPROACH

The best known of the theories based on consideration of consequences is **utilitarianism,** where the predicted consequences of a decision or action would be utility – the greatest good for the greatest number. In other words, that which would create the greatest benefit for everyone involved in the situation or, in some circumstances, society as a whole.

In this theory the end justifies the means. In other words, in its purest form (act-**utilitarianism**), so long as utility is achieved, it does not matter how it is done. Critics of this theory suggest that the means include deception, coercion or ignoring the needs of individuals, perhaps creating local misery to gain global benefit (Jones 2000). Some armed conflicts could be seen to be examples of this effect. To non-utilitarians this approach would seem immoral. A modified version, known as rule-**utilitarianism**, still requires the achievement of utility, but by more socially acceptable means. For instance, if society expects people to be honest, then lies and deceit would not be used to achieve utility.

The further up the management levels a midwife climbs, the more likely it is that at least rule-**utilitarianism** is employed. The reason for this approach is the nature of the job. Even a shift leader or ward manager has to consider the allocation of available resources, including staff, with a view to achieving the greatest benefit for all the women and babies. The remaining members of staff, however, may be in a better position to consider the needs of the individual women and babies. The more senior the manager, the more strategic the responsibilities, the more utilitarian the decisions and actions, whether related to childbearing women, babies or staff.

Another criticism of this approach is that it is impossible to be certain of the predicted outcomes of all decisions or actions. There might be many variables, particularly in complex situations, which could prevent the achievement of the intended consequences.

Any of the above approaches could be adopted by midwives to assist them in their decision making. Choosing an approach that best matches their normal values and their work setting (clinical, managerial, educational), plus being aware of the possible difficulties related to that approach, will probably ensure greater success. Having considered briefly the basic elements of these four approaches, it is important to see how they could be applied in practice. As screening has been used as an example earlier in the chapter, this topic will be continued in the scenario below.

APPLICATION OF ETHICAL APPROACHES

Scenario 7.1

Sarah is a 15-year-old girl who is at 17 weeks' gestation in her first pregnancy. She has already been booked and had a dating scan. Today she has attended your clinic for her appointment, with Pauline, her mother. You have explained to both of them about serum screening and anomaly scanning. Pauline immediately states that all screening tests should be carried out. She and Sarah's father will be the source of support for Sarah and her baby and she does not want the added burden of a baby with a disability.

Sarah, however, does not want the blood tests taken, nor does she want the anomaly scan. She is adamant that she will not have a termination of pregnancy (TOP) if an abnormality is discovered.

✎ Activity 7.3

Determine what action you should take – would you act in accordance with the wishes of Sarah or Pauline? Consider each of the four approaches previously discussed.

PRINCIPLES

If you choose to take the Principles approach, you will need to consider the four main principles of autonomy, beneficence, non-maleficence, and justice. You will need to consider what degree of autonomy Sarah is entitled to and your decisions must be just – not discriminatory with regard to her age. You are her advocate and need to consider what is of benefit to Sarah, not to her parents, and you need to prevent harm to her. The fact that she is a minor in age does not automatically mean that her mother can make decisions for her, although she may believe that she has this right. If Sarah is deemed legally competent, in accordance with the Fraser standard, known as **Gillick competence** (Gillick v. West Norfolk and Wisbech AHA 1986) and the Children Act 1989, then she can make decisions for herself (Jones and Jenkins 2004). Transferred into an ethical context, that means that if she appears to have thought about her options in a **rational** manner, then she is at liberty to make her own decisions, unless her decision puts her life at risk. In this case, Sarah appears to have given thought to her situation and articulated her views **rationally**, indicating that her autonomy should be respected. She also could be protected by the Human Rights Act 1998, probably under Article 8 regarding *private life and family*. As she is not old enough to marry, Article 12 related to the *right to marry and found a family* would not apply at this time.

With regard to benefit and harm, you need to consider how Sarah would benefit from anomaly screening. It might give her peace of mind to know that her fetus was normal but, unfortunately, screening cannot achieve this end result. The tests themselves do not prevent abnormality; also, they cannot give any guarantees that what has been screened for is not present, they only give a ratio of risk. It would not be of benefit for her to know if the result indicates a high risk, as she has stated quite clearly that she would not have a TOP. The main benefit that can be assumed relates to the mother and she is not the client, the one for whom you have a **duty of care**. Pauline would initially feel happier that the tests were done and she might exert less pressure on Sarah. However, she would have no guarantee that the baby would be free from abnormality. In addition, if the results indicated a high risk of abnormality, then Pauline would expect Sarah to undergo a TOP, which she says she does not want. Her attitude to Sarah through the rest of the pregnancy could create greater hardship for Sarah.

There appears to be no benefit for Sarah if she were to undergo the screening offered. On the contrary, it would appear that there is a reasonable risk of causing harm, especially as it has been well established that antenatal screening creates anxiety for many women, even when their views are not the same as Sarah's. It is possible that Pauline could create a situation of stress for Sarah, which could also be harmful, but your actions cannot be determined by the possible actions or desires of the parents.

VIRTUES

To use this approach, the midwife must possess the required virtues; a list of some suggested virtues has already been included in the brief description of the approach. It would appear that, directed by these virtues, the midwife must intuitively know what decisions to make in this situation, with the common good in mind (Velasquez and Andre 2003b). The common good would probably take account of the situation from the viewpoint of all the stakeholders: Sarah, her parents, the potential child, and possibly also society. This approach could be seen to have some common ground with utilitarianism, in that it is not only concern for the subject that is focused upon, but consideration of the whole picture. However, virtues would not automatically guide the decisions and actions for a utilitarian.

What would the genuinely honest, compassionate, fair and prudent midwife, who exhibits integrity, decide in this situation? If a virtuous midwife believes that much suffering can be caused by the birth of a disabled child into a family, then perhaps this belief may provide the substance and direction of the honesty, compassion and so on. Perhaps you might try to persuade Sarah to at least agree to the tests, to give some indication of the situation and possibly prepare herself and her family. However, you may believe that selective abortion for fetal abnormality is discriminatory, in which case, perhaps you would try to persuade Pauline that Sarah is making the right decision. If, as the virtuous midwife, you do not instinctively base your virtuous actions on your own beliefs, then presumably your decision must be to ensure that Sarah is competent and making her decision based on the necessary information and then support her.

DUTIES

In this approach, whichever form of **deontology** is followed, it is Sarah on whom the focus lies, not the significant others who might be considered when seeking either utility or the common good. As with any of the ethical approaches, the starting point, as expected in law, would be to determine whether or not Sarah was competent. If she is not competent then the mother would be able to make decisions for her. However, even if Pauline determines that the tests should be carried out, Sarah may physically prevent the taking of a blood sample and there is a limit as to how much force could be exerted, especially as the procedure is not required to save Sarah's life. If Sarah is considered to be **Gillick competent**, as indicated earlier, then she can make her own informed decisions.

If your ethical stance is Kantian, then you would focus on Sarah's autonomy. You would ensure that she has all the information that she requires to make her decision and you would act according to her wishes. If you felt that she had not had time to consider her options fully then you might suggest another appointment to give her more time. If you were assured that she had made an informed choice then you would decide to uphold her decision and inform Pauline accordingly.

If your stance was that of an intuitive pluralist, you would consider Ross's seven duties (1930), prioritising them according to the circumstances. Probably the duties of beneficence and non-maleficence would be at the top of your list, so your immediate concerns would relate to benefiting Sarah and preventing harm to her. Your decision would relate to the time in question, not to any future consequences of your decision; you would not be concerned with the possible outcome of the birth of a child with an abnormality, or a complaint from an angry parent that you ignored her wishes. As stated earlier with regard to the principles of beneficence and non-maleficence, deciding to undertake the tests against Sarah's will, based on her **rational** articulation, would be of no benefit and could be harmful.

Possibly the next duty that you would consider would be fidelity, which requires that you act in good faith towards Sarah, as your professional relationship is with her, not her mother. This duty would also include respect for autonomy, as discussed with regard to Kantianism. Justice would possibly be applied next and you would no doubt consider that Sarah should not be discriminated against because of her age. If she has shown herself to be competent and **rational**, then the fact that she just happens to be less than 16 years of age, when parental decisions might be accepted, should not be used to her detriment. The remaining three duties (reparation, gratitude, self-improvement) are less relevant to this case; therefore, less weight is given to their application.

CONSEQUENCES AND UTILITY

If the utilitarian approach is chosen, then the focus will be on the greatest benefit that can be achieved for the most people, according to the predicted consequences of your decisions. The people to be considered directly are Sarah, her parents and the potential person, currently the fetus. There is a broader, more indirect view, however, which relates to society and the perceived burden of a child born disabled and in need of indefinite support from many angles, including financial. An overall cost-benefit analysis would be conducted, with a view to determining which decision would result in more benefit than cost to the majority of the interested parties.

Supporting Sarah's autonomy and acting in accordance with her informed decisions would be seen to be of benefit to her. However, an impassionate assessment could suggest that, should the baby have an abnormality, Sarah's life could be unduly burdened, more so than might be expected by the birth of a baby with no known abnormalities. The burden would also extend to her parents, as they appear to be her source of support. Some people would believe that the burden could further extend to society, with the potential need to provide support and services for life. Undertaking the screening tests would give a ratio of risk of certain abnormalities that, although not precise and flawless, could give guidance as to any further advised action, such as diagnostic testing and possible TOP.

Acting in accordance with Pauline's wishes, therefore deciding to disregard Sarah's autonomy, would be **paternalistic**. It would also be somewhat dishonest, as you would have to state that Sarah was incompetent to make the decisions, thus requiring parental consent to be sought. However, if these costs could be predicted to be outweighed by the benefits – that is, appeasing Sarah's parents; reducing their anxiety if low-risk results are received; removing the burden of an abnormal child, to the family and society, by consenting to TOP if the results determine a high risk for abnormality, then such action would be seen to be morally correct.

The potential child is also affected by whatever decisions are made. Although a fetus has no rights in British law, it is a potential person and some people would wish to consider the possible consequences for it. Some of these people would determine that being born with an abnormality, which could lead to disability, would be a greater burden than benefit to that person. Others believe in the absolute principle that life itself has value and great benefit that outweighs

the burden created by disability (Miller 1996). When making the decision in this case, you could be swayed by your belief in this area. If you believe that being born with a potential disability would be a great burden, then you are more likely to support Pauline's stance.

Making predictions as to the potential consequences is not an exact science; it is based on presumption rather than fact. It could be that screening tests would give false-positive or false-negative results. Sarah could either go on to have a baby with an abnormality, when the risk had appeared low, or she could have a TOP based on a high-risk prediction, only to find that there was no abnormality. The effects of either outcome could be detrimental to Sarah and her family.

Taking a utilitarian stance when making decisions can be quite compelling. Most people, for most of the time, would like to make decisions that suit everyone. However, in reality, the more difficult the decision the more likely it is to find that it does not suit everyone. In midwifery, when considering settling for benefiting the majority, we must consider whether the person for whom we have a **duty of care** – the mother or the baby – will be a beneficiary or a cost bearer. If the latter is true, then perhaps this approach should be deemed to be inappropriate in this case.

As can be seen by the application of four of the common ethical approaches, any one of them could be appropriate. It depends on the stance of the individual making the decision or the onlookers who might judge it. What matters for consistency is that the same approach is used in similar situations (Velasquez and Andre 2003a). For instance, if there were four such cases in one month, it would be inconsistent – and therefore unethical – to use a different approach for each case. If it was felt that the duties approach was right in Sarah's situation, then the same approach should be used in the other three. It would be inappropriate, for instance, to use the utilitarian approach in one of the cases based on the fact that the mother was more compelling or manipulative.

The use of each of these ethical approaches involves subjectivity and, according to Round

(2001), their use in practice is not confirmed; rather, she suggests that it is the experience of the individual that influences their thinking. As there appears to be no moral approach or particular moral **value** that is essentially objective, some ethicists turn to ethical relativism in seeking solutions and making decisions (Seedhouse 1998).

ETHICAL RELATIVISM

While it is seen by most ethicists as preferable that consistency of approach is achieved, some ethicists believe that it is impossible to achieve consistency across societies, as there is no objective standard of truth (Seedhouse 1998). Their belief is based upon the variations in acceptability of a variety of practices, such as infanticide and certain forms of punishment, among others. In midwifery – and particularly in some parts of the United Kingdom – midwives are facing both moral and physical challenges related to female genital mutilation of young girls, which is an illegal practice in the UK. Regardless of the illegality of the practice, most people in our indigenous society would consider it to be immoral, abusive and therefore irrational, whatever the culture of the families concerned. Relativists, however, might suggest that, if such practices are the moral norm for that culture, then they should be accepted, as they are only comparatively irrational.

Those ethicists opposed to the principles of relativism, might use the argument that supporting a variety of moral norms within one society leads to inconsistency and, therefore, contradiction that is unsustainable. Others might suggest that effectively supporting practices because it suits that societal group prevents moral reform and improvement (Velasquez and Andre 2003a).

ETHICAL MODELS OR FRAMEWORKS

In an attempt to assist in the process of making ethical decisions, some ethicists have determined structured diagrammatic models or frameworks.

For instance, Seedhouse (1998) developed 'The Rings of Uncertainty' and 'The Ethical Grid'. However, structured, diagrammatic models do not appeal to everyone. Some people work best with a staged framework. One such framework is advocated by Velasquez and Andre (2003c) (see Figure 7.1).

This framework could assist with the varied situations in which midwives have to make decisions. It does not require adherence to one particular approach, in fact it encourages broader consideration and application, which could take account of the different levels of responsibility that midwives experience. Of course, as with any framework or model, it is not immediately helpful in emergency situations. However, for the truly reflective practitioner, the

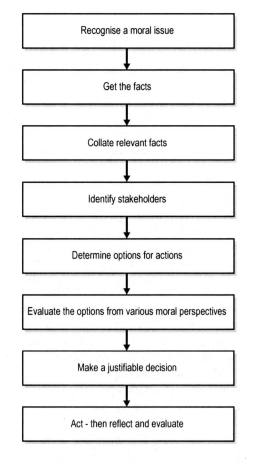

(based on Velasquez and Andre, 2003)

Figure 7.1 A staged framework. (Based on Velasquez M, Andre C 2003c Ethics and Virtue. www.scu.edu/ethics/practicing/decision/framework.html.)

framework could be applied in retrospect and the reflection and evaluation would assist the midwife when she next experiences a similar emergency situation.

SOURCES OF SUPPORT AND GUIDANCE FOR THE MIDWIFE

Further support for the midwife in developing ethical decision making can be found in the Code of Professional Conduct: standards for conduct, performance and ethics (NMC 2004a) and in the Midwives Rules and Standards (NMC 2004b). Supervisors of Midwives can also be approached for help or to debate the issues, as their role includes consideration and application of ethics and law (see Chapter 11). Also, it is important to have multi-professional discussions surrounding ethical **dilemmas** in practice; this can be achieved in a number of ways, including peer reflection on specific cases.

CONCLUSION

This chapter has considered four major ethical approaches to decision making and, with the aid of a scenario, those approaches were applied. Any one of the approaches could be deemed acceptable to some observers while unacceptable to others. Support for one approach above the rest has not been given, nor was it intended. Midwives should

familiarise themselves with the general approaches and utilise them according to the circumstances at the time; adherence to one particular theory or approach is not advocated (Beauchamp and Childress 2001). Midwives must remember that the woman, or the neonate, must be the central focus in the decision making process, regardless of the **values** of the midwife, which might be different from those of the woman or even different from those of the profession (Pritchard 1996). What is essential, however, is that they are consistent in their approach in similar settings to prevent contradiction, therefore, preventing discrimination and inequality.

KEY POINTS FOR BEST PRACTICE

- All professional decisions should be underpinned by ethical considerations.
- There can be conflict and dilemma in decision–making, but use of ethical approaches can assist in their resolution.
- The duty of care encompasses the need for ethical practice.
- There are various ethical approaches that may appeal to different people and be more suitable in different circumstances.
- The women and/or neonates must be the central focus of decision making.

References

Beauchamp TL, Childress JF 2001 Principles of Biomedical Ethics, 5th edition. Oxford University Press, New York.

Cioffi J, Markham R 1997 Clinical decision-making by midwives: managing case complexity. Journal of Advanced Nursing 25: 265–272.

Children Act 1989. HMSO, London.

Clouser HD, Gert B 1994 A Critique of Principlism. In: Gillon R, Lloyd A (eds), Principles of Health Care Ethics. John Wiley & Sons, Chichester.

Gillick v. West Norfolk and Wisbech AHA [1986] Crim LR 113 (HL).

Hanford L 1993 Ethics and disability. British Journal of Nursing 2(19): 979–982.

Human Rights Act 1998. The Stationery Office, London.

Jones SR 2000 Ethics in Midwifery, 2nd edition. Mosby, Edinburgh.

Jones SR, Jenkins R 2004 The Law and the Midwife, 2nd edition. Blackwell Publishing, Oxford.

Loughlin M 2002 Ethics, Management and Mythology. Radcliffe Medical Press, Oxford.

Miller P 1996 Ethical Issues in Neonatal Care. In: Frith L (ed), Ethics and Midwifery. Butterworth Heinemann, Oxford, pp. 123–139.

Nursing and Midwifery Council (NMC) 2004a Code of Professional Conduct: standards for conduct, performance and ethics. NMC, London.

Nursing and Midwifery Council (NMC) 2004b Midwives Rules and Standards. NMC, London.

Re A (minors) (conjoined twins: separation) [2000] 4 All ER 961, [2000]10 LLR Med 425 (CA).

Round A 2001 Introduction to clinical reasoning. Journal of Evaluation in Clinical Practice 7(2): 109–117.

Pritchard J 1996 Ethical decision-making and the positive use of codes. In: Frith L (ed), Ethics and Midwifery. Butterworth Heinemann, Oxford, pp. 189–204.

Ross WD 1930 The Right and the Good. Clarendon Press, Oxford.

Seedhouse D 1998 Ethics. The Heart of Healthcare, 2nd edition. John Wiley & Sons, Chichester.

Velasquez M, Andre C 2003a Consistency and Ethics. www.scu.edu/ethics/practicing/decision/framework.html.

Velasquez M, Andre C 2003b Ethics and Virtue. www.scu.edu/ethics/practicing/decision/framework.html.

Velasquez M, Andre C 2003c Thinking Ethically: A Framework for Moral Decision Making. www.scu.edu/ethics/practicing/decision/framework.html.

Further Reading

Jones SR 2000 Ethics in Midwifery, 2nd edition. Mosby, Edinburgh.
This book provides more grounding in ethics and its application to everyday midwifery practice than this chapter alone can give.

Jones SR, Jenkins R 2004 The Law and the Midwife, 2nd edition. Blackwell Publishing, Oxford.
It is important to have an understanding of the legal principles within which you have to make decisions. This book sets out the expectations through three main routes of accountability: the profession, civil law and employment.

Nursing and Midwifery Council (NMC) 2004 Code of Professional Conduct: Standards for Conduct, Performance and Ethics. NMC, London.
It is very important that you know the content of this document very well. It provides very clear principles on which to base your decision making, which will assist to remain ethical and legal in your practice.

Seedhouse D 1998 Ethics. The Heart of Healthcare, 2nd edition. John Wiley & Sons, Chichester.
This book is particularly useful if you wish to consider the diagrammatic models and contrast their use with the staged framework indicated in this chapter.

Velasquez M, Andre C 2003 Thinking Ethically: A Framework for Moral Decision Making. www.scu.edu/ethics/practicing/decision/framework.html.
It is worth accessing the information on this website that provides expansion of the Staged Framework constructed towards the end of the chapter.

Chapter 8

Making Management Decisions

Vicky Tinsley

OVERVIEW

How decisions are made is very dependent on the context in which the decision-makers find themselves. Decision making is therefore likely to follow different pathways depending on how political, structural, personal and organisational frameworks are formed. This chapter initially presents a background to the National Health Service (NHS) reforming the quality of leadership techniques for effective management decision making, and then examines certain tools that managers may use to aid the decision-making process, using examples from practice. The final part of the chapter discusses the development and use of clinical guidelines and the importance of applying the knowledge gained from personal experiences of management decisions in order to learn from the process and consequently effect change in the work place. Activities for the reader to undertake are also included in the chapter, providing an opportunity to apply the theoretical principles presented.

BACKGROUND

The New NHS: Modern and Dependable (Department of Health [DoH] 1997) was one of the first acts of the incoming Labour Government. This document immediately swept away what was known as the 'internal market' and General Practitioner (GP) fund-holding. Le Grand et al. (1998) reported that these aspects had both failed to deliver efficiency gains and were also highly unpopular with staff and the public alike, for creating inequalities in access to care. In their place, the notion of a new NHS was to be reinforced.

Gillam (2001) suggested that there was renewed emphasis on improving health and ensuring equity in relation to service provision. Issues of quality in service delivery were to be addressed through the creation of clinical governance structures and increased accountability to patients and Local Health communities. The NHS Plan: A Plan For Investment A Plan For Reform (DoH 2000a) can be seen as a coherent attempt to develop, refine and implement the modernising agenda of the 1997 White Paper.

The NHS Plan (DoH 2000a) set out an ambitious vision for healthcare provision into the 21st century, with services to be designed around the client, being responsive to their needs and evaluation. This meant setting national standards, including the introduction of National Service Frameworks (NSF) in areas such as cancer care, diabetic services, maternity services, giving high-quality services, breaking down old-fashioned demarcations between professional groups, and using modern methods to provide care when and where it is needed. In 2002, further substantial funding was announced in the Budget to support these initiatives.

One of the drivers of the decision-making processes is accountability. In spite of rhetoric to the contrary, the underlying reason for the introduction of both general management and planned markets into the public sector was doubtless to drive down costs and expert stronger financial control over the seemingly bottomless pit of healthcare expenditure.

A central component of current health policy was that there was to be a direct link between increasing the participation of more NHS staff in the decision-making process and the successful implementation of key policy changes. In particular, enhanced clinical performance is directly associated with the development of more open and efficient communication systems.

There were further organisational changes under way that had an effect on midwifery practice and the maternity care environment. The major structural change introduced to deliver these policy goals were the Primary Care Groups (PCGs), which then evolved into Primary Care Trusts (PCTs). In terms of the role of midwives, the PCTs support the expanded role of the midwife and the development of leadership in midwifery. Midwives have corporate, advisory and provider roles within PCTs. A typical PCT may cover 100,000 people and could have a budget of £70 million; larger PCTs may have budgets up to £150 million. Clinical and Corporate Governance structures also have a remit to ensure that PCTs have the required leadership and managerial capacity in midwifery, nursing and health visiting.

The role of manager has been shifted from one of energising control to one that is dealing with change. This shift of emphasis means that managers need to develop different skills from those that sufficed in a fairly static bureaucracy. Repeated restructuring of the workplace has broken down longstanding relationships that were usually of a supervisor/subordinate kind. While a move away from a rule-bound role culture is to be welcomed, for a number of reasons these changes can lead to isolation of the various groups which in turn need to be managed.

Changes in the configuration of NHS Trusts have favoured a move away from the hierarchical management structure to one that is flattened. This means increased management responsibility, and control has been given to clinically based midwives for which a wide range of knowledge, skills and expertise are required. This means that those already holding a management position take on a bigger span of control. The advantages for midwives working in such a structure, as Andrews (1994) points out, is that it gives them more opportunity for local autonomy and decision-making (see Chapter 1). It is not always necessary for midwives to go right to the top of the organisation, as decisions can be made and implemented at a lower level. However, for some midwifery managers this means that, as they take on more management control, they will become responsible for an increasing number of midwives. To stay on top of the job, a wide range of skills and techniques are now required.

Now undertake the following activities highlighted in Activity 8.1.

Activity 8.1   Points for Thought and Discussion

- Define the management structure within the organisation you work.
- Identify the key decision-makers in the organisation: what is your influence on decision making?
- Identify the members of the Trust Board and their areas of speciality/background.
- Define how you would contact them should there be a particular issue you wanted to raise.
- Define how clinical guidelines are developed in your organisation.
- What do these guidelines tell you about the values of your organisation?
- Identify how you can ensure that the needs of women remain central to the goals of the organisation.

QUALITIES OF LEADERSHIP

Cross (1996) states that effective managers are also effective leaders, and that management and leadership are intertwined. Although there are some distinctions between management and leadership theories, in reality the difference is less clear. Managers can be taught management skills, but for the growth of leadership, managers must first possess basic personal qualities and a belief in the fundamental values of human behaviour. Transforming leadership is about empowering others to be their own leaders. The model illustrated in

Figure 8.1 shows the multi-faceted role of the competent midwifery leader.

Heller and Hindle (1998) comment that a simple definition for a manager is someone who gets things done through the activities of others, and yet the meaning of management is mostly misunderstood. This is not surprising, because management is not a unitary concept but a highly complex process. The over-riding managerial role is that of decision making. Managers need to consider other aspects of their job that may or may not facilitate the way the maternity services perform. By breaking down the traditional management process into components, different roles and responsibilities can be identified. *Communication* is a theme, which runs through each component, emphasising the importance and power of effective communication in management. Tourish and Mulholland (1997) also suggested that a *sound knowledge of management theories* facilitate an understanding of why managers and workers behave and function in the way they do. Katz and Kahn (1978) state that to perform effectively, managers require *technical*, *human* and *conceptual skills*, but the balance of technical and conceptual skills will vary according to the manager's level and position in the organisation. Human skills remain constant at all levels, taking up

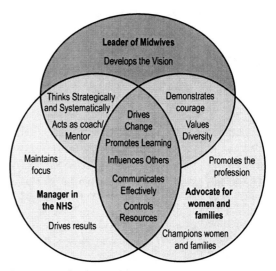

Figure 8.1   The multi-faceted role of the competent midwifery leader.

most of the manager's time. The role and sphere of influence managers have within the organisation is illustrated in Table 8.1.

It is the task and constant preoccupation of a manager to have a good understanding of policy as it relates to his or her unit, to understand the external relations of the unit, and to have a view on the direction of development of the unit in the context of the development of the organisation. This gives the manager a frame of reference for decision making, which is used to respond to requests from the staff for guidance and direction. Thus, the manager by decision making is likely to be the leading agent of evolutionary change, but this role is greatly facilitated by the quality of the questions and suggestions, which form the main vehicle for change agency, by the staff.

Hayward et al. (1999) argue that a distinguishing feature of decision making is that it occurs at a discrete moment in time: a choice is made on the information available and the other options available are discarded. The timing of the choice is important, neither too early before adequate consideration has been given and valid options identified, nor too late so that good options have lapsed with the passage of time or progress of work is delayed. Effective decision making is about formulating events, bringing about results, and modelling the future. Ineffective decision making thwarts change, and making reactive decisions deals with the short term only. Escalation and entrapment may result from short-planned decisions and cause decision makers to become trapped in losing courses of action. In other words, the decision-maker needs to continue despite obstacles, persisting and refusing to accept defeat.

DEFINING DECISIONS

A decision is a choice between a variety of alternatives, and a decision-maker is whoever makes such a choice. Hayward et al. (1999) states that a decision can be made instantly but more often involves the decision-maker in a process of identification, analysis, assessment, choice, and planning. Benner (1984) comments that to arrive at a decision, a manager must define the purpose of the action, list the options available, choose between the options, and then turn the choice into action. Decisions and the process of decision-making are fundamental to all management processes – just as they are to everyday life.

Heller and Hindle (1998) believe that a decision is a judgement or choice between two or

Table 8.1   The Manager's Role and Sphere of Influence

Who	How	Type of Decision
Trust Board Level	• The final decision-making body of the organisation. • Responsible for clinical/corporate agenda	• PCT assets such as land/hospital sale • Closure of a clinical area • Financial recovery plan
Executive Professional Committee	Sub Committee of Board clinical representative elected to the committee combined with managers	• Recommendations made to the Trust Board
Directorate Level	• Combination of the following structure in each organisation. e.g. Medical Director, Director of Service, Support Services, IT, Finance, Personnel, Clinical Manager.	• Future direction of Maternity Services • Implementation of National documents. • Dependent on Commissioner's services.

more alternatives, and arises in an infinite number of situations from the resolution of challenges or difficulties encountered, to the implementation of a course of action. Managers of people, by definition, must be decision-makers. However many situations occur when the decision has been made already, i.e. Trust Board Level decision but the manager can still influence these decisions.

DIFFICULTIES WITH DECISION MAKING

Decision making really always begins with a challenging or difficult situation, but in reality these do not suddenly appear. They may just become more of a reality and more urgent for attention. Often, the midwifery manager or the organisation may not even be aware that a difficult situation in the workplace exists because the staff keep it to themselves or do not recognise it as a problem as it is just the 'norm'. However, challenging or difficult situations are often ignored until they become a crisis, as they are not a priority.

DIFFICULTY WITH DETERMINING CHALLENGING/DIFFICULT SITUATIONS

The ability to recognise and then define a challenging or difficult situation depends on having the correct information. This is often not easy to obtain and sometimes crucial data may even be unobtainable. Frequently information about challenging situations is restricted to gossip and rumour, and staff may be reluctant to give details to managers. Information gathering is only part of attempting to determine the difficulties. Being able to interpret the information is critical, but if the information is incomplete then mistakes in decision making can be made. It cannot always be taken for granted that a challenging situation is always understood. Sometimes those who make decisions do not really understand the difficulties, and occasionally they are not even interested in solving it. There may not be an overall solution that fits all situations that prove to be a challenge. Furthermore, not all difficult and challenging situations that need a decision are actually resolvable. Decision making is neither simple, nor rational.

CATEGORISING DECISIONS

The various types of decision that a manager has to make include routine, emergency, strategic, and operational. Many decisions are *routine*: the same circumstances recur, and when they arise a proven course of action is chosen. Some situations, however, are without precedent – the decision is made on the spot or as events unfold. This is *emergency* decision making, and this can take up most of a manager's time. The most demanding form of decision making involves *strategic* choices: deciding on aims and objectives, and converting these into specific plans, or sub-decisions is a manager's most important task. *Operational* decisions – especially those concerned with difficulties with people (including hiring and firing) – require particularly sensitive handling.

UNDERSTANDING RISKS

Most decisions involve an element of risk, though some are less risky than others. Sometimes, even when theoretical options exist, their disadvantages are so great that there is no real alternative. This may arise from an original ill-informed decision. For example, it could be decided to halt the ongoing project, but only at the risk of immediate financial collapse. Therefore, to retreat is riskier. Also, managers need to remember to watch for knock-on risks. Reducing staff may seem a safe decision, but not if it risks deterioration in customer service, jeopardises safety and causes a rise in complaints.

DECISION MAKING IN A DEMOCRATIC CONTEXT

Managers can make decisions:

* *Autocratically*, with or without consultation.
* *Democratically*, where subordinates have an equal say in the decision.
* *By consensus*, where all parties discuss until they agree on the decision.

Within the organisational settings, managers usually reach some kind of balance between these different decision-making styles, depending on the organisational culture, personal style and the particular decision that needs making. However, Young (2002) argues that there is a pressure in large bureaucratic organisations such as the NHS to impose decisions on subordinates. There are two reasons that this appears inappropriate and unacceptable. First, as citizens of a democratic public sector, employees value concepts such as equality and choice. Second, professionals value their own autonomy and expect some degree of consultation and involvement in the decision-making process.

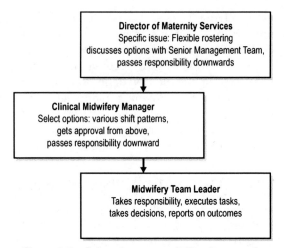

Figure 8.2   Delegating responsibility downwards.

DELEGATING DECISIONS

Although the manager is responsible for making decisions to delegate activities to others, the accountability rests with the person to whom the activity was delegated. In particularly sensitive areas, it is important that she or he oversees the delegation process. This is an ideal opportunity to try to build up the confidence of the people to whom the decision was delegated. It is essential to maintain a two-way flow of information, and to encourage people to develop their own initiative. Any decision should only be rejected after a full discussion with the person concerned.

PUSHING DECISIONS DOWN

When analysing responsibilities, it is clear that those closest to the point of decision making should also take the decisions. For example, changes in off-duty rota, changes in team composition, and so on (see Figure 8.2). Information at the sharp end is likely to be specific and up to date. Those who have to live with decisions should participate in them. Sending decisions upwards can cause delay: the more hierarchical layers there are, the greater the potential for delays. Pushing decisions down pays off in speed and efficiency, though delegates need to be monitored and

supported to develop their decision-making skills.

MAKING FAST DECISIONS

It is important to be able to assess whether a decision can be made quickly or whether it can wait. For example, the manager needs to prevent a knee-jerk reaction to a complaint that will change the whole service for the benefit of one client, the result being a short-term gain with long-term consequences. Rather, the manager will have to decide on the spot whether to grant the concession in order to keep the client's goodwill. Good decision-makers often do make instant decisions, but the long-term implications will have to be assessed.

AVOIDING PITFALLS

Consulting others, in some cases, can have more disadvantages than advantages. First, there is the time factor: the more people consulted – however qualified they are to comment – the longer the decision-making process will take. Furthermore, the greater number of people approached, the higher the chances of confusion occurring due to contradictory opinions. Second, the manager may lose control over the entire process if too many people become involved. In order to avoid these pitfalls, the manager needs to keep a tight grip on proceedings, and limit the number of opinions to those that are really essential. Token or partial consultation does not succeed. The manager who reverses a decision after hearing the contrary views of a meeting is strong rather than weak.

GROUP DECISION MAKING

Groups sometimes make decisions, and often groups are consulted – either formally or informally – over decisions that have been proposed for local and national changes. Handy (1993) believes that effective groups – be they problem-solving or producing – are the ones that set themselves standards and have a maintenance programme in practice. He contends that groups where the leader does not get the group to set and adopt standards, will be satisfied at the lowest level as far as decision making is concerned.

There is also the question of whether groups should make decisions at all, because of the way they behave and function. When a group makes a decision, it may not be totally reliable and will depend on what process was adopted to agree the decision. Drummond (1991) argues that effective decision making requires all views to be articulated and debated seriously. Everyone in the group should be encouraged to contribute, and all members should properly consider each of the contributions. The group decision-making process can range from consensus to coercion. If a leader presupposes power, this can distort the decision-making process. Usually groups are counter-productive when decisions require speed and concentration, but can be effective for generating ideas and providing views and comments.

It has been shown in experimental studies (Handy 1993) that groups who attack a problem systematically perform better than those who muddle through, or evolve. The performance of the group will be influenced by the kind of approach they adopt, and how each member is encouraged to participate.

TOOLS TO ASSIST DECISION MAKING

To reach a sound decision, the manager needs to analyse all the relevant facts. There are several analytical tools that are both useful and simple to employ. Use of analysis leads to strong conclusions, and therefore good strategic decision making.

SWOT ANALYSIS

Walton (1995) suggests that in many circumstances, a SWOT (Strengths, Weaknesses, Opportunities and Threats) analysis is helpful. This technique, which was developed at Harvard Business School and is often used in a marketing context, is frequently used in NHS organisations to achieve change. A SWOT analysis helps to clarify the larger picture around the circumstances of change, and aids the formulation of the arguments. The process is often illustrated in the format illustrated in Table 8.2.

The strengths and weaknesses relate to the internal environment of the organisation or team; for example, the situation of an individual having to introduce the change. The opportunities and threats are concerned with the external environment, for example, the reaction of the team when the change is being introduced.

A SWOT analysis works best when the participants (representatives of the team, organisation, or relevant stakeholders) allow their thoughts to emerge, and a note is made of anything and everything that comes to mind when considering the situation – no matter how bizarre it may seem. The ideas created from

Table 8.2 SWOT Analysis

STRENGTHS	WEAKNESSES
OPPORTUNITIES	THREATS

From: Walton M 1995 Management and Managing: Leadership in the NHS, 2nd edition. Stanley Thornes Ltd, Cheltenham, p. 217.

this process can be ordered later when the flow of thoughts has come to an end, and a clear list can be written down. This method of 'brain-storming' frequently generates ideas and actions in a broader context, which other approaches might otherwise curb.

A useful point to consider when drawing up a SWOT analysis is to address each section separately and to list the issues in each of these different sections. It is essential to keep the lists separate so that the issues are not mixed up. It is possible for some items to appear in two lists (e.g. something may be both a threat and a potential opportunity).

The outcome of a SWOT analysis is to identify the main issues that need to be addressed as a clear action plan. There will be elements in the SWOT analysis that cannot be influenced, and this is to be expected. An action plan is likely to be successful if it concentrates on the areas (people and actions) that can be influenced and is discussed with all that are concerned.

Now undertake Activity 8.2.

Activity 8.2

In order to reduce its direct budget costs for the coming financial year for the maternity services, the Trust Board have informed you, as the Director of Midwifery Services, that the annual birth figures will need to increase.

By undertaking a SWOT analysis, consider the Strengths and Weaknesses that currently exist within your service and those Opportunities and external Threats that may influence the decisions you make to address this mandate.

This may also include identifying the strengths and weaknesses of neighbouring maternity services that also serve the needs of the local population.

COMMITMENT CHARTS

Another management tool to assist a manager's decision making is described by Ham (2002). The identification of the relevant stakeholders who may help or hinder the achievement of change, and of their potential positive participation in working out in detail the precise action plan required, is an important step. However, the subsequent action plan will only actually work if the support and commitment from these individuals (and others who may be affected) is obtained. One way of identifying people's commitments to change is to follow the step identified in Box 8.1.

Showing this process diagrammatically can help to clarify the level of commitment and the change required. The level of commitment can be judged using the following scale for each individual, as shown in Figure 8.3.

Case Scenario 8.1

The unit is working towards the Baby Friendly Global Award. Following on from an audit, there is one ward team that appears to be having difficulties, so the manager has used a commitment chart (see Table 8.3) to try and identify the problems and then develop an action plan.

The commitment chart in Table 8.3 illustrates how the midwives' current position and where he or she needs to be for the change to occur can be shown. The difference between the two gives a rough measure of the work that may need to be

Box 8.1 Commitment to Making Decisions that Influence Change

- List the key stakeholders who are required to support the change.
- Select from the list those stakeholders whose support is essential; they are the 'critical mass' of support.
- Assess the current level of commitment from each individual within this 'critical mass'.
- For each individual, assess what the desired future level of commitment should be for the successful implementation of the proposed change. This step should highlight who should be involved.

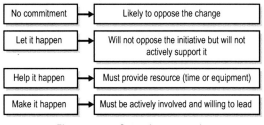

Figure 8.3 Commitment scale.

Table 8.3 Commitment Chart

Midwife	No Commitment	Let it Happen	Help it Happen	Make it Happen
1		x ⇒	⇒	O
2				x O
3		x ⇒	O	
4	x	⇒	O	
5			x O	
6	⇒	x	⇒	O
7			x ⇒	O
8		x O		
9	x ⇒		⇒ O	
10			O	x ⇐

KEY: O = Required level of commitment;
X = Current level of commitment.

done in order to obtain the necessary commitment from the midwives. In this chart, midwives 5 and 7 hold the required position, and midwives 1 and 6 have the furthest to move. Midwife 10 represents an individual who, although committed, may adversely affect the process if involved; for example, their interpersonal skills may put off others whose commitment is vital. Midwife 2 is most likely to act as 'champion for change', as the current and required level of commitment coincide and fall in the 'making it happen' column. It is helpful if that champion is perceived to have the respect of others within the team organisation. Using the principles identified above in relation to commitment in the workplace, now undertake Activity 8.3.

Activity 8.3

* Consider your decision to introduce a new practice within the maternity unit in which you work.
* Identify key midwives who can influence this decision, either positively or negatively.
* Draft a commitment chart as in Table 8.3 so as to determine where you perceive each midwife fits in according to their commitment to the innovation.
* Develop an action plan as to how you will address any challenges to you implementing this innovation.

INFORMATION TECHNOLOGY

Information technology is increasing the pace of change in healthcare, and is rapidly becoming an important medium for patient information. It gives access to decision-making processes and provides information amassed by government agencies, foundations and academic institutions. Global accessibility to the Internet is increasing the potential awareness of clients to all available options for treatment.

HANDLING INFORMATION

Before feeding information into the decision-making process, the manager must organise and check it thoroughly, never taking anything for granted. Reports from outside consultants or internal sources should come properly organised, with all conclusions clearly stated at the beginning of the report, supporting data arranged in a logical order, and all relevant information gathered into logical sections.

Ball et al. (2003), in their Birthrate Plus Framework, describe the principles of planning data collection, collation and analysis within the complexity and variations of maternity service delivery throughout different areas of the United Kingdom (UK). Ball et al. (2003) reported that it became apparent that, without expert guidance, many managers and midwives would be unable to achieve a robust and reliable outcome to compare current establishments and inform future planning initiatives. This enables comparisons of, for example, midwife per category of care, patterns of work, and case mix, together with an initial examination of ratios of the numbers of:

* Hospital births per whole time equivalent midwife per annum.
* Home births per whole time equivalent midwife per annum.
* Case load-base birth per whole time equivalent midwife per annum.

This gives the manager the information to be able to take decisions about the workforce, with the key questions being:

* Is the workforce being managed in the correct way?
* Are the midwives in the right place at the right time with an appropriate workload?

THE USE OF CLINICAL GUIDELINES IN MANAGEMENT DECISIONS

According to Ham (2002), guidelines are statements that have been systematically developed in order to assist practitioner and client decisions about appropriate healthcare for specific clinical circumstances. Since the 1990s, there has been a marked increase in the use of guidelines in clinical practice to the extent they are now a familiar part of routine healthcare, which Ham (2002) attributes to a number of factors including:

* rising healthcare costs, fuelled by an increase in patient demand.
* more expensive medical technologies.
* an ageing problem.
* variations in the delivery of healthcare in hospital and community services.
* geographical variations in healthcare, possible due to over- or under-use of services.

NATIONAL CLINICAL GUIDELINES

These are the guidelines that have been developed by clinicians and sponsored by the relevant professional body or bodies according to nationally agreed standards. Over a period of time, national guidelines will either be produced by, or have the formal approval of, the National Institute for Clinical Excellence. The topics chosen for such guidelines are, in part, determined by national priorities for clinical governance; for example, October (2003) saw the launch of the Ante-Natal Care for Low Risk Women (National Institute for Clinical Excellence [NICE] 2003).

LOCAL CLINICAL GUIDELINES

These are guidelines that have been issued at a local level, for example Trust, PCTs, strategic health authority or practice guidelines. These may or may not have been derived from national guidelines. In addition, these are guidelines that have been produced to reflect local health care needs and priorities where there may not be any national guidelines available. In some cases there may be a number of guidelines for the same condition (e.g. diabetes).

BENEFITS AND LIMITATIONS OF GUIDELINES

The development of good practice guidelines and Clinical Governance reporting structures embraces the general principles of risk management to:

* Inform the decision making of clinicians, clients and managers.
* Change practice where appropriate.
* Monitor outcomes.

It is important to view guidelines as tools for helping the clinician, in conjunction with women, to make the most appropriate decisions on clinical care based on the best available evidence. However, it is not appropriate for clinicians to follow blindly the steps in guidelines, setting aside their clinical expertise and experience without reference to the woman in front of them. Guidelines are there to provide information on the expected outcomes of treatment in the majority of cases. However, clients do vary in their responses to treatment, and it is in these situations that clinical acumen takes over from guidelines. Having stated this, guidelines do provide a general reference point for the minimum expected standards of care.

The main benefit of guidelines is to improve the quality of care to clients by improving health outcome through the promotion of effective interventions and discouraging ineffective care. The result ideally is to reduce morbidity and mortality and to improve the quality of life. The principal limitation of guidelines is that the recommendations could be wrong if poorly constructed. It is important to note that clinicians are expected to follow the guidelines produced by NICE, and if this is not done a careful note should be made in the client's record explaining why this is so.

DEVELOPMENT OF GUIDELINES

Many health professionals feel threatened by the concept of guidelines. Ham (2002) suggests that the use of guidelines inhibits the clinical freedom of the individual practitioner and the decision making of managers and does not add to the quality of care of clients. However, national and local guidelines do assist the managers' decision making in ensuring consistency to the quality of care and saves time in not re-inventing the wheel over decision-making issues. Simply implementing guidelines cannot ensure that practice is always safe. If practitioners are expected to follow standards, protocols and guidelines, there are a number of important lessons that can be learned (as indicated by DoH 2000b) in Box 8.2.

This calls for a manager who can support the organisation in learning how to learn as well as being a change agent, initiating and adopting change that builds on the organisations capacity to maximise its potential for effective healthcare.

CONCLUSION

Ham (2002) suggests that less hierarchical approaches would lead to great involvement in decision-making. Recent changes in the NHS have led to flatter and fewer hierarchical structures. Ham (2002) also claims that

Box 8.2

- All guidelines for practice are properly ratified, and those individuals who are responsible for ratifying them are aware of their ethical and legal duties for clients, staff and to the organisation.
- The responsibility also means understanding the contemporary evidence, knowledge, skills and competence available as a benchmark on which to base these guidelines.
- Guidelines are regularly updated to keep abreast with policy, professional and technical developments and research including new technology and skills.
- The knowledge base from which the guidelines are developed is supported by a range of appropriate acceptable evidence.
- Practitioners do not make decisions solely on the basis of clinical or policy guidelines but must exercise their professional judgements.
- The organisation learns from its mistakes, analyses the whole complex system of care to identify gaps in the service and provides the 'organisation with a memory' that is not reliant on one person.

Source: DoH 2000b.

these changes have led to decentralised decision-making and that there is now a greater degree of employee involvement in decision making that correlates with improved employee commitment. Modernising the health service requires fundamental and radical change at all levels of service. New organisational structures are demanding different accountabilities and altered management relationships.

The people providing the care have the potential to inform and to shape strategic and operational decisions. To be able to rise to this challenge and participate in re-shaping and improving services, midwives and other professionals need to be equipped to manage complexity, uncertainty, ambiguity and intractability of problems, which exist in a concentration and is not found in other service industries. The NHS is often characterised by difficulties/problems that complicate the decision-making process and make absolute or perfect solutions intangible. No single approach or strategy will fit all the situations that arise. Practitioners and managers must be skilled in selecting the right tools for the particular circumstances that face them. They also need to recognise that the world of healthcare is at best chaotic and messy and that a muddling through, or incremental approach to decision making is probably the best it gets.

There appear to be two common misconceptions about decision making. The first is that this is a rational and scientific process (see Chapter 4), and the second is that a decision is an incredibly complex activity involving an interaction between the individual and the whole organisation. Effective decision making is about formulating events, bringing about results and shaping the future. Moreover, Drummond (1991) believes that as well as action, the future can also be shaped by 'inaction or decisive-inaction', which stems from so-called 'non-decision making' that can deliberately thwart change.

The manager's decision-making style will change depending on the decision required, and the urgency of making that decision. In an ideal world, the manager would involve all appropriate members of staff in all decisions. Unfortunately, due to the constraints on manager and staff this is not always practical or realistic. Post-mortems into management – like those in medicine – usually follow a disaster, whilst successful decision-making techniques are often neglected. Few decisions stand completely alone, and in most cases one decision leads to another to form a continual process of decision making, feedback and analysis. However, it is as important to know why decisions succeed as to explain why decisions may fail. The exact circumstance of the decision and its action plan may never reoccur, but a successful methodology could hold important lessons for the future.

Currently, the complexity of decision making has been compounded by the pace of modernising reform which has created an environment that demands more woman-centred services, and has complex lines of accountability and responsibility. The consequence of a flatter organisation and the increasing emphasis on inter-organisational partnership working needs new roles that have a greater emphasis on strong interpersonal relationships and political sophistication which sustains pressure to innovate continuously to improve service delivery and quality. These reforms are of course to be applauded; however, there also needs to be recognition of the toll that this can take on sometime struggling, over-stretched healthcare workers. In response, leadership development and management training needs to understand how people change, adapt and apply learning about decision making in the workplace. Practitioners must be able to transfer their learning back into organisations in ways to develop organisational memory and deliver change. Support is needed to enable people to put new ideas into practice. It is not enough simply to have the knowledge without it being applied when making management decisions. In addition, the use of reflection to assess the learning that has arisen from personal experiences of management decisions is important to procure successful decision making in future practice (see Chapter 10). This may sometimes mean dealing with failure as well as success, but failure may provide some of the most powerful learning opportunities.

KEY POINTS FOR BEST PRACTICE

- Decision making is a highly complex process and is compounded by the pace of modernising reform.

- Managers should facilitate appropriate decision making, using all available information.

- Managers need to be consistent in their decision–making approaches.

- Decision making should be made at the correct level of decision-making authority.

- The nature of challenging/difficult situations determine the nature of decision making.

- Managers in position must make decisions and not prevaricate!

- All decisions have a consequence, and managers must always be aware

- of the consequences of their decision making.

- Reflecting on management decision-making, both successes and failures should be seen as a learning opportunity that can effect future decision making.

References

Andrews A 1994 Managing your Manager. Nursing Standard 8(31): 49–54.

Ball J, Bennett B, Washbook M, Webster F 2003 Birthrate Plus Programme: a basis for staffing standards. British Journal of Midwifery 11(5): 264–266.

Benner P 1984 From Novice to Expert: Excellence and Power in Clinical Nursing. Addison-Wesley, Melor Park, California.

Cross RE 1996 Midwives and Managers. A handbook. Book for Midwives Press Publication, Cheshire.

Department of Health (DoH) 1997 The New NHS: Modern and Dependable. The Stationery Office, London.

Department of Health (DoH) 2000a The NHS Plan: A Plan for Investment – a Plan for Reform. The Stationery Office, London.

Department of Health (DoH) 2000b An Organisation with a Memory. Report of an Expert Group on Learning from Adverse Events in the NHS. The Stationery Office, London.

Drummond H 1991 Effective Decision Making. Ludlow, Kogan, Page Ltd, London.

Gillam S 2001 Primary Care Evolving Policy. In: Gillam S, Brooks F (eds), New Beginnings Towards Patient and Public Involvement in Primary Health Care. Kings Fund, London.

Ham C 2002 Health Policy in Britain. The Politics and Organisations of the NHS, 3rd edition. Macmillan Press, University of Birmingham.

Handy C 1993 Understanding Organisation: The New Face of the NHS. Langham Group UK, Ltd, Harlow Essex.

Hayward J, Rosen R, Dewar S 1999 Thin on the ground. Health Service Journal 26: 26–27.

Heller R, Hindle T 1998 Making Decisions. Dorling Kindersley Ltd, London.

Katz D, Kahn R 1978 The Social Psychology of Organisations. Wiley, Chichester.

Le Grand J, Mays N, Mulligan J (eds) 1998 Learning for the NHS

internal market: A review of the evidence. Kings Fund, London.

Midwifery Leadership Competency Model. The National Nursing Leadership Programme. NHS Modernisation Agency, Manchester.

National Institute for Clinical Excellence (NICE) 2003 Antenatal Care: Routine Care for the Healthy Pregnant Woman. Clinical Guidelines 6, London National Collaborating Centre for Women's and Children's Health. NICE, London.

Tourish D, Mulholland J 1997 Communication between Nurses and Nurse Managers: a case study from the NHS Trust. Journal of Nursing Management 5: 25–36.

Walton M 1995 Management and Managing: Leadership in the NHS, 2nd edition. Stanley Thornes Ltd, Cheltenham.

Young A 2002 The Political Context of Decision Making. Managing and Implementing Decisions in Health Care. Ballière Tindall, Harcourt Publishers, London.

Further Reading

Pickering S, Thompson J 2003 Clinical Governance and Best Value. Meeting The Modernisation Agenda. Churchill Livingstone, London.

This book covers many issues that influence decisions within healthcare management. Topics include clinical governance requirements and achieving change.

This text can enhance understanding of the factors that influence midwifery managers' decisions for care provision.

Covey S 1999 7 Habits of Highly Effective People. Free Press.
This book is written by a management consultant and is widely recommended for management courses. It provides accessible advice for achieving effective *behaviour. Many healthcare managers strive to make decisions within this framework.*

Tappen RM Weiss SA Whitehead DK 1998 Essentials of Nursing Leadership and Management. FA Davis Co, Philadelphia.
This book gives a step by step guide to managing change and other management activities, such as dealing with conflict and motivating others.

Chapter 9

Helping Women to Make Their Own Decisions

Pauline Cooke

INTRODUCTION

Human decision making, particularly within the politically sensitive context of healthcare, has been described as one of the most complex of activities (Elwyn and Edwards 2001). It therefore follows that helping women make their own decisions in pregnancy and childbirth, while arguably a fundamental aspect of midwifery practice, is no easy task. Levy (1999a: 118) comments: "Midwives are frequently in the position of helping women in their care to make choices that may have far-reaching effects on their lives, as well as upon their babies and families, when the outcome of that choice is uncertain."

The concept of decision making from the woman's perspective is inextricably linked to that of exercising and making informed choices. There is substantial evidence to indicate that involvement in decisions helps achieve a positive birth experience and improved psychological outcomes (Green et al. 1990a, Lavender et al. 1999). However, it would appear that there is a large minority of maternity care users who do not feel involved in decision making. A study in the UK in 1996/7 found that 52% of women said they were fully involved in all decisions about their pregnancy and 54% in decisions during labour and birth (Wyke et al. 2001).

If involvement in decisions during pregnancy and childbirth is important to women, it seems worthwhile considering how midwives can facilitate this activity. This chapter will set the context for decision making both at an organisational level and at the individual level. It will analyse the factors which may influence women and suggest some helps and hindrances before discussing the knowledge, skills and attitudes of a midwife engaged in facilitating decision making. Finally, a framework for working alongside women will be suggested, illustrated by an exemplar.

THE DECISION-MAKING CONTEXT

ORGANISATIONAL CONTEXT

The National Health Service (NHS) has seen a growing amount of changing healthcare policy over the past 10–15 years. Changing Childbirth (DoH 1993), in response to the Winterton Report (House of Commons Health Committee 1992) provided a potential catalyst for change in maternity care provision. It promoted woman-centredness and the importance of involvement in decision making. It remains open to debate how far-reaching this policy was to effect real change, but it nonetheless spearheaded the introduction of popular concepts such as choice, user involvement and partnership working into the language of the NHS.

The House of Commons Health Committee returned its scrutiny to the maternity services in 2003 and recommended that the Department of Health ensured that "… women are given a genuine and informed choice, and not the illusion of choice" (p. 32) which some women reported was the current situation. It also recognised that involvement in decision making was the "… key to a positive experience of childbirth" (p. 75). Just a few months later, the Government engaged in a major consultation exercise on how best to improve choice, responsiveness and equity in the NHS. The strategy paper published in December 2003 confirmed the commitment to 'real' rather than 'theoretical' choice where "information and the power of personal preference (is) extended to the many" (p. 3). Indeed, the consultation exercise found that 76% of those who

replied identified greater involvement in decision making as being important and the strategy paper has adopted the term 'shared decision making', where users are engaged and informed, as the way forward.

In its response to the House of Commons Health Committee, the Government (2004) affirmed its commitment to improving and providing choice for women; faced with the recommendation of recasting maternity services to the advantage of both women and their carers, it lays responsibility on the Children's National Service Framework (NSF) (DoH 2004) as "… likely to emphasise the centrality of women and their babies in maternity care" (p. 43).

User involvement in healthcare is now a political imperative. The NHS Plan (DoH 2000) has this as a central theme in its proposed changes and emphasises more information, more choice and increased involvement in decision making. The Children's NSF (DoH 2004) had a sub-group devoted to user involvement. The Commission for Patient and Public Involvement has been set up by Government as an advisory and review body, managing the performance of the new Patient and Public Involvement forums which will review the effectiveness of trusts in responding to the user's voice.

In its emphasis on user involvement, the Government often describes the relationship between healthcare professionals and patients as a partnership (DoH 2002, 2003a, NHS Executive 1996) and lays considerable weight on the nature of such relationships: "Patients have told us time and time again that it is relationships and communication at every level which make the difference." (DoH 2003a: 68).

WOMEN'S DECISIONS

What is the nature of the relationship between a woman and her midwife, and how can this facilitate decision making? This relationship is often characterised as a partnership. Kirkham (2000) draws a continuum of a woman's engagement with the maternity services from professional control, where the service is unknown at the one extreme, through an interim position of negotiation where relationships with individual midwives may develop, to partnerships and women-centred care at the other extreme. The balance of power increasingly tips towards the woman. Pairman (2000) also identifies partnership as a way of describing the health professional/client relationship which is egalitarian rather than hierarchical. In reality, each partnership is unique and inevitably some partnerships will be more equal than others.

There needs to be collaboration and sharing of ideas, perspectives and information. While midwives may know more about the physiological changes in pregnancy, women can contribute their own experience of this, their knowledge of their own bodies, their values and their preferences; each partner brings expertise to the relationship. The term 'mutuality' is a way of describing the notion of both sides of the partnership contributing to and benefiting from mutual respect and the opportunity to learn from each other. Pairman (2000: 224) describes this as a "... reciprocal relationship ... that is mutually empowering", but partnership is also about midwives sharing themselves and being "... with women" (Kirkham 2000).

The issue of trust is also of significance. Trust is about developing confidence in one another so that the woman feels safe and secure (Anderson 2000). This is facilitated by a relationship built up over time with a known midwife. Women may feel vulnerable during pregnancy and birth, and the issue of trust may be even more relevant in situations of risk or emergency where there may be little time to discuss or negotiate. A woman may leave decisions to the midwife's judgement if she trusts her (Blix-Lindstrom et al. 2004, Harding 2000, Levy 1999a).

Encouraging choice and involvement in decision making is justified by appealing to the ethical principle of autonomy, which has been described as the central and possibly most important principle in midwifery (Pritchard 1996). A successful partnership is one where both the woman and her midwife exercise autonomy: the woman in terms of her right to

exercise choice and self-determination, and her midwife in terms of her professional role and ability to make decisions, independent of others, in uncomplicated pregnancy and birth. The issue is fundamentally about personal power to make decisions and is linked to ideas of control. But autonomy has to be followed by responsibility (see Chapter 1).

The International Code of Ethics for Midwives (ICM 1999) supports the midwife's role in promoting the woman's acceptance of responsibility for the outcome of her choices. The midwife is also an accountable practitioner, but the idea of sharing responsibility for decisions may be a complex one to grapple with. Pairman and Gulliland (2003: 229) summarise these ideas thus:

"In the midwifery partnership model both the woman and the midwife retain responsibility for their individual decisions and the midwife as a health professional is expected to apply her professional knowledge base. For both the woman and the midwife the concept of partnership is premised on their autonomy, their ability and their right to make decisions together ... and to take responsibility for those decisions."

FACTORS THAT INFLUENCE WOMEN

There are a number of factors that may influence women in their decision making and are important for midwives to analyse and understand their impact.

PREFERENCE FOR DECISION-MAKING STYLE

Charles et al. (1999a) describe a conceptual framework for decision making in healthcare, and identify three approaches: the paternalistic; the shared; and the informed decision making approach. In later work, Elwyn and Charles (2001) develop this thinking around the three approaches in terms of information exchange, deliberation and decision.

In the paternalistic approach, the information exchange is largely one way from professional to patient, and the amount communicated is the minimum that is legally required. The deliberation and discussion of the information is by the professional alone or with colleagues, and the patient's preferences are either not sought or are over-ridden. The decision about treatment is made entirely by the professional.

In the shared decision-making approach, the information exchange is two-way with interaction; the professional shares all the information which is relevant, for example options, benefits and risks, and the patient shares personal information about lifestyle, preferences and values. The deliberation is between each other and potentially others, including family and friends. Negotiation and support are important to reach a consensus.

In the informed approach, the information exchange is largely one way from professional to patient, with the professional acting as a research transfer agent, responsible for communicating options, benefits and risks. The deliberation is by the patient either alone or with family and friends as information is weighed and an informed decision is reached without the professional expressing opinions or preferences.

O'Cathain et al. (2002a) developed their research on women's perceptions of informed choice and used a model to elicit women's decision-making style, with the options ranging from making the choice themselves, through three grades of shared decision making, to leaving the health professional to make the decision. O'Cathain et al. (2002a) asked women which role they preferred when making decisions during pregnancy, and the majority (83%) wanted some form of shared decision making, whereas 14% wanted to make the final choice (informed decision making) and only 3% wanted to leave the decision to the health professional (paternalistic decision making).

Women clearly do have a preference for decision making, but this may not be fixed and may differ according to the type of decision or when it is made, for example, when in pain or distress. Establishing women's preferences for decision making may be of importance in

facilitating this activity and could be a useful tool for discussion during pregnancy and birth. In everyday practice, decision making is likely to combine elements of these approaches and a degree of sensitivity and flexibility is necessary when dealing with women of differing needs. Preferences for decision making are summarised in Figure 9.1.

SOCIAL AND CULTURAL ISSUES

It is all too easy to fall into the trap of stereotyping women regarding their likely involvement in decision making. How often are negative comments heard or made about women with clearly thought out birth plans? The study of Green et al. (1990b) contributes much to our thinking and, contrary to popular stereotyping, found that those women who were less educated did not want to hand over all control to the staff, but did experience less involvement in decision making than the well-educated middle-class women. Similarly, O'Cathain et al. (2002a) found in their antenatal sample that more women from manual occupations, those who left full-time education before reaching the age of 18 years and multiparous women, preferred not to share decision making with health professionals and were located at either end of the model described in Figure 9.1.

Stapleton et al. (2002a) found that many women in antenatal consultations – particularly those who were young and/or poor – remained silent and spoke very little, usually only in response to direct questions from either the midwife or the doctor. In addition, the assumed correlation, made by many midwives, between a woman's social class and her knowledge base was not supported. Stereotypical assumptions had a direct and negative impact on the care of materially deprived women (Kirkham et al. 2002). In the Choice consultation, some of the strongest messages from disadvantaged groups were about their search for greater influence and control over decisions. The Government have stated the importance, therefore, of ensuring that arrangements for supporting choice including

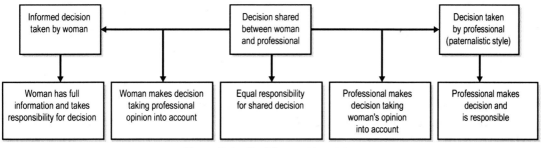

Figure 9.1   Decision-making styles.

information and support for shared decision making respond to the "... full diversity of community needs" (DoH 2003a: 52).

Many midwives work in large cities with shifting populations and different language groups. Whether or not a woman has sufficient grasp of English or access to female interpreters will undoubtedly affect her involvement in decision making because the "... complexity of assumptions and meaning embedded in any language does not readily translate into the factual data on which contemporary evidence based approaches rely." (Stapleton 1997: 61).

ACCESS TO INFORMATION

Shapiro et al. (1983), in their study on information control, found that women from lower socio-economic groups, although desiring more information, obtained less than did women from higher groups. In terms of written information available, *The Pregnancy Book* (DoH 2003b) is the free publication given to all first-time mothers, but significantly this is only available in English and Welsh and not in large print, braille or on audiotape. *You're Pregnant* are local maternity guides recently produced by the Department of Health in association with Dr. Foster, outlining the range of local services available, and the Department is examining the feasibility of producing these and *The Pregnancy Book* in different languages (Government Response 2004).

Other written information available may include local trust leaflets. Each unit will have its own mechanism for scrutinising the quality

of written information. Users play a vital role in contributing to these leaflets and tools such as DISCERN (Charnock 1998) can be helpful in evaluating the quality of health information.

Midwives Information and Resource Service (MIDIRS) have produced an updated revision of the Informed Choice leaflets. These take the form of paired leaflets for health professionals and for women. Some trusts have purchased these leaflets, but in terms of their success in promoting informed choice in everyday practice, a randomised controlled trial found – disappointingly – that they were not effective (O'Cathain et al. 2002b). Some of the possible reasons for this will be examined later.

Women access information from many different sources including radio, television, magazines (containing a mixture of horror and miracle stories), books, family and friends, health professionals and other organisations. Some access the Internet, which displays a wealth of information about pregnancy and birth. This information may lack balance, accuracy or evidence. Some of the new initiatives for information outlined in the Choice Strategy (DoH 2003a) may have potential for improving access and increasing involvement in decision making. HealthSpace, which will be linked to the electronic NHS health record in 2006, will be a facility for individuals to record their preferences and will contain a birth plan; and a national NHS Direct digital TV service will provide health information which may reach less affluent groups of the population.

Although access to information may be one factor in determining women's involvement in decision making, it cannot stand independently of support and opportunities to discuss the information with a midwife.

POWER

"The supposedly woman-centred rhetoric of choice and informed consent assumes a level playing field on which women can state their wishes." (Edwards 2000: 74). This is not necessarily the reality in everyday practice, where ruts and molehills may mar the playing field. Levy's study (1999a) highlighted many issues of power and how this affected women's involvement in decision making. Women assumed power over decision making if they felt confident of their understanding of the information. This was dependent upon perceptions of their status within the system. Women were reluctant to expose themselves in terms of their decision making if midwives appeared to impose their own choices, and therefore 'played the game' and went along with the midwife, not revealing their intentions, for example, not to breastfeed.

Another issue concerns what Stapleton and colleagues (2002a) term 'the continuum of engagement between the woman and her midwife'. At the end of the continuum there may be a pre-determined agenda set by the midwife, largely to instruct the woman; at the other end, the agenda is shared and a more egalitarian approach is used where strategies are employed by the midwife to enable the woman to be involved and voice her concerns. If the midwife controls the agenda of what may be discussed, she is acting as a gatekeeper not only of information but also of what decisions may be made as a consequence (Levy 1999c). In this situation, women are unlikely to perceive their involvement as welcome or significant.

Finally, how women view midwives and other health professionals may affect their involvement in decision making. The 'professional knows best' may be a less common belief but it is still powerful. Levy's (1999b) study illustrates this point where women often seemed to regard midwives as dominant, possessing knowledge and authority to direct the choices they made. Essentially, this is about the balance of power between a woman's autonomy and her perceptions of the professional's authority.

PERCEPTIONS OF RISK AND SAFETY

Our perceptions of risk and safety are inseparable from how we broadly view the world and the kind of society we want to live in. It is therefore important that these perceptions are placed in the social and cultural context of everyday life (Stapleton 1997, Bellaby 2001). There is a direct relationship between these perceptions and decision making in pregnancy and childbirth.

Hope (1996: 4) commented that: ". . . individuals differ both in what they value and in their propensity to take risks." No human activity is completely free from risk, and it is up to the individual to decide what constitutes an acceptable risk. Women in pregnancy have their own standards by which they evaluate risk, and these probably reflect their values, education, social class and culture (Saxell 2000). Women faced with the same situation, for example, carriage of group B *Streptococcus*, with access to the same information provided by the same midwife, may take different decisions concerning intrapartum antibiotics (Cooke 2003).

It is also important how a woman defines safety. This may differ from how the health professional defines it. Midwives and doctors tend to have narrow, short-term definitions of safety in terms of mortality and morbidity. They may ignore the wider view, involving factors such as emotional and psychological well-being (DoH 1993). Health professionals may also view safety as entirely a matter for their own judgement, defining what constitutes an acceptable level of risk (Kirkham 2000). In this situation, the woman is encouraged to put herself totally in the hands of the professional, and her involvement in decision making is greatly reduced.

The home birth debate is an area where issues of risk and safety may feature. Edwards (2000), in her study of women planning homebirths, found evidence of women choosing homebirth to avoid risk in terms of inappropriate intervention. However, women's attempts to decrease risk could be viewed by health professionals as increasing it. When these definitions of risk and safety diverged, women did not feel supported in decision making. Edwards (2000: 50), comments: "If women are encouraged by health professionals to conceptualise risk superficially in terms of the 'safety of the baby' then … women will usually prioritise this over any need they may have, including that of birthing in an environment which they perceive as safe and supportive."

FACTORS THAT HELP OR HINDER DECISION MAKING

In thinking about facilitating women to make decisions there will always be factors which work with us, and others which seem to work against us, in achieving this goal. First, we will consider the factors that help.

ENGAGING WITH UNCERTAINTY

The notion of uncertainty may seem, at first sight, contrary to the concept of decision making, but much of the literature on choice and decision making alludes to it. Leap (2000) coins the term 'embracing uncertainty' and states that no amount of screening or information can provide complete certainty for the woman. Kirkham (2000) states that midwifery is about living with uncertainty and helping women to do so. Evidence-based guidelines and quality standards cannot completely control childbearing and overcome uncertainty. Holmes-Rovner et al. (2001: 276) predict a future where health professionals and patients come to "… embrace uncertainty and love difficult choices." Their debate is based on the premise that evidence-based medicine, with its emphasis on effectiveness of treatment, does not always reduce the uncertainty of healthcare outcomes, particularly when there are equally feasible treatment options available.

One way of helping women engage with uncertainty could be in preparing them to keep an open mind about options. This may mitigate

against the current re-emphasis on birth plans (DoH 2003a), but as Leap (2000) contends, the journey through pregnancy and birth includes uncharted landscapes for which there can be no planning.

KEEPING UP TO DATE WITH INFORMATION

This seems essential if we are to help women come to decisions, but it can be daunting. There are evidence-based leaflets such as those produced by MIDIRS and evidence-based guidelines, for example, those produced by the National Institute for Clinical Excellence (NICE), which are written both for women and for professionals. Not every midwife has the necessary skills of literature searching and critical appraisal of evidence, so such leaflets and guidelines can be invaluable.

However, care does need to be exercised in our use of them. Stapleton and colleagues (2002a,b,c) found that the mere distribution of leaflets to women did not facilitate decision making, and suggested they should be used as a starting point for discussion, in response to individual need, and not a statement of fact.

USER GROUPS AND PATIENT PUBLIC INVOLVEMENT FORUMS

In many ways the potential of user groups to challenge the status quo in maternity care has not been fully realised. Now that user involvement is accorded high status and deemed essential in the planning of maternity services, there may well be opportunities for joint working in the provision of information and the promotion of choice and decision making in education and practice which should be explored.

Having identified factors that help decision making, attention will now be given to factors that hinder.

ACCEPTANCE OF THE 'ROUTINE'

Health professionals and women may accept many tests and practices as a routine part of being pregnant or in labour. This may inhibit involvement in decision making. Levy's study (1999d) illustrates this in that blood tests for grouping, haemoglobin estimation and rubella status were accepted unquestioningly as routine, and that fetal screening tests, although 'optional extras' were presented as extensions of the routine. The House of Commons Health Committee (2003) drew attention to this very issue by stating their belief that simply making tests available is not an extension of choice; rather, it may inhibit rational choice and encourage higher levels of intervention.

RESOURCE ISSUES

Stapleton et al. (2002b) report on the extra time required to share complex information with women generally unused to active participation in antenatal care. Pressures of time restricted the information that midwives gave and limited the interaction with women. The limited time available was given disproportionately to middle-class women who were most able to access information independently (Kirkham et al. 2002). The impression was of midwives so pressured that women were not given time to speak and were 'robbed' of their voice (Stapleton et al. 2002a). Levy (1999a,e) found a similar theme with midwives needing to limit the amount of time in interacting with women at booking interviews, whilst trying to appear not to do so.

In other healthcare settings, Charles et al. (1999b) also draw attention to the way that time may act as a disincentive for doctors to explore and respond to patient's preferences in the process of making decisions. Capacity is another issue that may create a barrier to helping women in decision making. This has been recognised by Government (DoH 2003a).

ORGANISATIONAL CULTURE AND POWER STRUCTURES

It would seem that the greatest barrier is organisational culture and its hierarchical power structures. There is some evidence that, where midwives provide continuity of carer, the trusting relationship which develops as a result generally enables women to initiate conversations, ask questions at a deeper level and articulate wishes and concerns (Stapleton 2002a, Harding 2000, Pairman 2000, Freeman et al. 2004). This may have something to do with such relationships reducing imbalances in power and with the midwife's primary allegiance to the woman rather than the institution that employs her.

Stapleton and colleagues (2002c) describe a hierarchy of power that was evident in the units they studied, with obstetricians at the top, midwives and other health professionals in the middle and pregnant women at the bottom. These inequalities in power and status are a potent force that works against shared decision making. It may result in obstetricians defining the norms of practice and, as a result, the choices that are available or acceptable.

In such a culture of inequality, there are limited opportunities for midwives to act autonomously. This can result in midwives steering women to the 'right' choices in order to protect the status quo (Stapleton et al. 2002b, Levy 1999d,e). Such behaviour only serves to reinforce the power structure. Essentially, midwives tend to treat women as they themselves are treated and ". . . disempowered midwives disempower women." (Edwards 2000: 80).

Although efforts have been made in recent years to define a social model of birth (Walsh and Newburn 2002), the medical model remains strong in many consultant units and has a pervading influence on the organisational culture. Stapleton and colleagues (2002b,c) found that information giving largely supported technological intervention where its risks were minimised and its potential harm was withheld, for example, fetal monitoring. Fear of blame by the power-holders ensured that midwives recommended a 'right' choice, for example, Caesarean section for breech presentation and reduced the potential of making a 'wrong' choice.

Finally, the language that midwives use in their interactions with women indicates where the balance of power lies and reflects personal attitudes (Stapleton 1997). A popular concept in the language of shared decision making and informed choice is that of empowerment. However, Leap (2000) maintains that none of us can empower another person because power is taken, not given. The phrase 'giving informed choice' betrays professional control and needs careful reflection on the meaning it conveys. The danger is in adopting the rhetoric about involvement, partnership and informed choice but exhibiting behaviour and conversational strategies that merely ensure compliance with our professional agenda (Stapleton et al. 2002a,b; O'Cathain et al. 2002a).

KNOWLEDGE, SKILLS AND ATTITUDES

Several authors have highlighted the problem of reducing shared decision making to a stripped down set of tasks, skills or behaviour which fail to encompass the complexity of blending information giving with the degree of support necessary in practice (Greenhalgh 1999, Towle and Godolphin 1999, Elwyn and Charles 2001). Key competencies are presented in Box 9.1.

How can a midwife develop these attitudes, knowledge and skills? One way would be to seek out role models and tap into their expertise. Resources such as the MIDIRS Informed Choice Learning Zone have interactive modules designed to develop skills for facilitating informed choice. However, skills such as these are not always valued. There is evidence that midwives who practise them may be marginalized and alienated by colleagues (Stapleton et al. 2002e, Levy 1999e).

FRAMEWORK FOR DECISION MAKING

There are a number of published frameworks for shared decision making in medicine (Towle and Godolphin 1999, 2001, Elwyn and Charles

---

Box 9.1 Key Competencies for Facilitating Women's Decisions

Attitudes
- Willingness to engage in a collaborative partnership approach.
- Recognition of a woman's autonomous right to make decisions for herself.
- Respect for the values, beliefs and decisions of a woman which may be different from ours.
- Willingness to relinquish professional power.

Knowledge
- Knowledge of evidence including the benefits and risks of particular options.
- Understanding of ethical theories underpinning decision making.
- An understanding of the midwife's professional responsibility and accountability.

Skills
- Self-awareness of potential personal bias.
- Presenting information impartially.
- Listening and responding to the woman's concerns.
- Questioning and the use of open questions to elicit the woman's preferences and check her understanding.
- Supporting women in their decisions, even though we may not agree with them.
- Advocacy and identifying with women whose choices may be unconventional.
- Handling conflict concerning decisions.
- Reflection and analysis of the process and outcome of decision making.

2001), and a model for evidence-based practice in midwifery (Page 2000), which has been particularly influential in the development of these ideas. It is important to recognise that decision making for women does not necessarily follow a logical or linear pattern (Stapleton 1997), and sometimes decisions need to be made quickly in labour without much time for discussion or recourse to published information.

Box 9.2 Decision-Making Processes

- Establish the woman's preferred decision-making style
- Explore the woman's values and beliefs
- Access information
- Discuss, deliberate and decide
- Reflection

However, a sequence of decision making processes is presented in Box 9.2. The sequence of events may alter according to the requirements of a situation.

This framework is illustrated by Case scenario 9.1, in which the names have been changed to protect anonymity. Grammatically, the first person is used because this case study is based on personal experience.

CONCLUSIONS

The concept of involvement and partnership in decision making is not only an important principle of current NHS policy, but it also has the potential to transform both the individual experience of women and the maternity services which provide care. While the rhetoric is often used, the promotion of involvement in decision making is not yet widely accepted and the current structure of our maternity services with their inherent power hierarchies form the biggest barrier to change. Midwifery skills, attitudes and knowledge can all be developed, but a coherent strategic initiative is necessary to address professional control and power imbalance. Alliances with users, representative of our local populations will be important, as will structuring services around meaningful, collaborative relationships with women. Models of care need to be thoughtfully developed which advantage both women and midwives leading to mutual trust and reciprocity. Countries such as New Zealand, with its partnership model should give us hope and inspire us. Are we ready for the challenge?

Case Scenario 9.1

Lisa was a 30-year-old school nurse, married to Robert. I had been her midwife for her two previous pregnancies.

- Explore the woman's values and beliefs

Lisa rang me one evening to tell me she was pregnant again and asked if I would be her midwife. At the outset, Lisa told me two things which were important to her: first, that she try for a vaginal birth, and second, that she breastfeed. Her previous babies had been born by elective Caesarean section, and although she attempted to breastfeed, she had changed to bottle feeding at 3–4 weeks. Her main reason for wanting a vaginal birth was that she would recover more quickly and be able to look after her boys, including driving them to school and playgroup.

This was also likely to be her last pregnancy and there was a sense of wanting to experience labour and birth. Robert fully supported her in her wishes.

- Establish the woman's preferred decision-making style

Lisa wanted to be fully involved in all decisions, but told me that she valued my opinions and that of a sympathetic obstetrician.

- Access information

In terms of Lisa's history, her first baby had presented by the breech for most of the pregnancy. She had declined an external cephalic version and opted for a Caesarean section at 38 weeks. The baby was admitted to the neonatal unit for a few hours with transient tachypnoea. In her second pregnancy, Lisa ruptured her membranes at 34 weeks and at 39 weeks, and requested a Caesarean section having been in hospital for so long.

Lisa was healthy with no significant medical or social problems. Her previous babies had weighed just over 3 kg, and this baby was growing well and of average size.

Other sources of information included the published literature on vaginal birth after Caesarean (VBAC). This included the National Sentinel Caesarean Section Audit (Thomas and Paranjothy 2001) which found an overall VBAC rate of 33% in England and Wales.

The draft NICE guideline on Caesarean section reported that there has been no randomised controlled trial comparing elective repeat Caesarean section with VBAC, but observational studies suggest that uterine rupture is rare – about 18 per 10,000 in women with a previous Caesarean section. Rosen and Dickinson (1990) in their meta-analysis reported an absolute risk of uterine rupture of 0–28 per 1000 for women who underwent VBAC. There is less evidence for women undergoing VBAC after two previous Caesarean sections. Phelan et al. (1989), in a prospective study in the United States of 1088 women with two previous Caesarean sections, found that 46% of them attempted VBAC, with 69% of them being successful. The rate of uterine dehiscence was 1.8% in those who attempted VBAC. This was a similar finding to another study (Flamm et al. 1994) which found the risks of uterine rupture to be 1.8% with two previous Caesareans versus 0.6% with one. Enkin et al's conclusion (1990) was that the available evidence does not suggest that a woman with more than one previous Caesarean section should be treated any differently from the woman with just one.

At 34 weeks I saw Lisa and Robert together with a consultant obstetric colleague known for his open consideration of VBAC. This colleague had asked to see Lisa's previous notes, and there was no adverse comment about the lower segment. The obstetrician's opinion was that it was 'reasonable' to try for a VBAC avoiding prostaglandins and syntocinon and not ignoring signs of an obstructed labour.

- Discuss, deliberate and decide

This was ongoing throughout Lisa's pregnancy. In terms of the framing effect, the obstetrician probably emphasised the risks of VBAC, while checking out her resolve.

Lisa and Robert clearly understood the small risk of uterine rupture and that in very rare cases, it may endanger both her and her baby's life. I may have emphasised the benefits as a counterbalance. There was no doubt that this was an 'unconventional' choice but there was no need for advocacy as a clear plan was written in the notes and both she and I were aware of our responsibilities.

The plan we agreed was that Lisa would need to go into spontaneous labour at term and ideally remain upright and mobile to encourage steady progress. She would try to avoid an epidural, and I would carefully listen to the fetal heart for any bradycardia, which may indicate a problem. On admission to hospital, hopefully not until in established labour, blood would be taken and serum saved in the event of an emergency Caesarean section and blood transfusion proving necessary.

- Reflection

Lisa went into labour at 41 weeks after a membrane sweep the day before. I saw her at home mid-morning when she was relaxed and doing some ironing! She was contracting mildly every 5–10 minutes, her membranes were intact, and the fetal heart accelerated after a contraction. By mid-afternoon, having been mobilising all morning, she was contracting more strongly but still at the same frequency. She requested a vaginal examination which showed her cervix to be 3 cm dilated, fully effaced, and thick with the vertex 2 cm above the spines. She was encouraged by these findings and glad to be in labour. The plan was to continue at home, and I would return when the contractions became stronger and more frequent.

Lisa called me that evening when her contractions were much stronger and we made a plan to meet at the hospital. I could hear her as she arrived with Robert and she opted fairly quickly for an epidural. Thankfully, it seemed to have no effect on the strength and frequency of her contractions which by now were three to four every 10 minutes, and strong. She remained mobile until successive top-ups dictated otherwise and the continuous cardiotocograph since epidural administration remained reassuring throughout her labour.

By early morning, Lisa's cervix was fully dilated with the vertex in an occipito-anterior position and at the spines. After about 1½ hours of pushing with little descent, Lisa was exhausted and requesting help. A ventouse cup was used to assist her to give birth to her 3.9-kg baby girl, who was born in excellent condition.

Lisa transferred home from the labour ward after just a few hours, and I continued her care post-natally. She breastfed successfully, and when I asked her permission to use this story, she asked me to include that she only stopped at 9½ months because the baby seemed to want to!

It is an understatement to say that Lisa was delighted in having a successful VBAC. She often told me during our post-natal appointments that she felt completely different about herself and that her 'head was clearer'. She recovered quickly and was driving the boys to school and playgroup after 2 weeks. Her self-esteem and sense of achievement was high, and this has remained so throughout this first year. The benefit was mutual, and I certainly learned from the whole situation in terms of shared decision making with each of us having responsibility. The final decision was hers, but I was responsible for exercising professional judgement and ensuring that I would recognise a problem early and act on it. Another benefit for me was in collaborating with obstetric colleagues, and this has led to a number of other successful VBACs.

KEY POINTS FOR BEST PRACTICE

- Involvement in decisions by women helps achieve a positive birth experience and improves psychological outcomes.

- Government policy promotes choice, involvement in decision making and increased information.

- Decision making is facilitated by reciprocal partnerships between women and midwives, characterised by collaboration, trust, autonomy and responsibility.

- Women may vary in their preference for involvement in decision making, and are influenced by social and cultural issues, access to information, issues of power and perceptions of risk and safety.

- Facilitating decision making is helped by an approach which encourages engaging with uncertainty, keeping up to date with information and user involvement in the provision of information and the promotion of choice.

- Hindrances to decision making include acceptance of the routine, resource issues and the organisational culture.

- A framework for decision making includes establishing the woman's preferred decision making style, exploring her values and beliefs, accessing information, discussing, deliberating and deciding and finally, reflecting.

References

Anderson T 2000 Feeling safe enough to let go: the relationship between a woman and her midwife during the second stage of labour. In: Kirkham M (ed), The Midwife–Mother Relationship. Macmillan Press, Hampshire, pp. 92–119.

Bellaby P 2001 Evidence and risk: the sociology of healthcare grappling with knowledge and uncertainty. In: Edwards A, Elwyn G (eds), Evidence-based Patient Choice: Inevitable or Impossible? Oxford University Press, Oxford, pp. 78–94.

Blix-Lindstrom S, Christensson K, Johansson E 2004 Women's satisfaction with decision-making related to labour. Midwifery 20(1): 104–112.

Charles C, Gafni A, Whelan T 1999a Decision making in the professional–patient encounter: revisiting the shared treatment decision making model. Social Science and Medicine 49: 651–661.

Charles C, Whelan T, Gafni A 1999b What do we mean by partnership in making decisions about treatment? British Medical Journal 319(7212): 780–782.

Charnock D 1998 The DISCERN Handbook for Consumer Health Information on Treatment Choices. Radcliffe Medical Press, Oxford.

Cooke P 2003 Difficult decisions: group B streptococcus and intrapartum antibiotics. In: Wickham S (ed), Midwifery: Best Practice. Books for Midwives, Edinburgh, pp. 16–19.

Department of Health 1993 Changing Childbirth Part 1: Report of the expert maternity group. HMSO, London.

Department of Health 2000 The NHS Plan. The Stationery Office, London.

Department of Health 2002 Learning from Bristol: The Department of Health's response to the report of the public inquiry into children's heart surgery at the Bristol Royal Infirmary 1984–1995. Department of Health, London.

Department of Health 2003a Building on the Best. Choice, responsiveness and equity in the NHS. The Stationery Office, London.

Department of Health 2003b The Pregnancy Book. DoH, London.

Department of Health 2004 National Service Framework for Children, Young People and Maternity Services: core standards. DoH, London.

Edwards NP 2000 Women planning home births: their own views on their relationships with midwives. In: Kirkham M (ed), The Midwife–Mother Relationship. Macmillan Press, Hampshire, pp. 55–91.

Elwyn G, Charles C 2001 Shared decision making: the principles and the competences. In: Edwards A, Elwyn G (eds), Evidence-based Patient Choice: Inevitable or Impossible? Oxford University Press, Oxford, pp. 118–143.

Elwyn G, Edwards A 2001 Evidence-based patient choice? In: Edwards A, Elwyn G (eds), Evidence-based Patient Choice: Inevitable or Impossible? Oxford University Press, Oxford, pp. 3–18.

Enkin M, Keirse MJNC, Neilson J, et al. 1990 A Guide to Effective Care in Pregnancy and Childbirth, 3rd edition. Oxford University Press, Oxford.

Flamm B, Goings J, Yunbao L, et al. 1994 Elective repeat caesarean delivery versus trial of labour: a prospective multicentre study. Obstetrics and Gynecology 83: 927–932.

Freeman LM, Timperley H, Adair V 2004 Partnership in midwifery care in New Zealand. Midwifery 20(1): 2–14.

Government response to the House of Commons Health Committee Reports. Fourth report of session 2002-3 Provision of Maternity Services, Eighth report of session 2002-3 Inequalities in Access to Maternity Services and Ninth report of session 2002-3 Choice in Maternity Services 2004 Cm6140. The Stationery Office, London.

Green JM, Coupland VA, Kitzinger JV 1990a Expectations, experiences and psychological outcomes of childbirth: a prospective study of 825 women. Birth 17: 15–24.

Green JM, Kitzinger JV Coupland VA 1990b Stereotypes of childbearing women: a look at some evidence. Midwifery 6(3): 125–132.

Greenhalgh T 1999 Commentary: competencies for informed shared decision making. British Medical Journal 319(7212): 770.

Harding D 2000 Making choices in childbirth. In: Page LA (ed), The New Midwifery: science and sensitivity in practice. Churchill Livingstone, Edinburgh, pp. 71–85.

Holmes-Rovner M, Llewellyn-Thomas H, Elwyn G 2001 Moving to the mainstream. In: Edwards A, Elwyn G (eds), Evidence-based Patient Choice: Inevitable or Impossible? Oxford University Press, Oxford, pp. 270–288.

Hope T 1996 Evidence-based Patient Choice. Kings Fund Publishing, London.

House of Commons Health Committee 1992 Second Report, Maternity Services, Vol. 1. HMSO, London.

House of Commons Health Committee 2003 Fourth report of session 2002-3 Provision of Maternity Services, Eighth report of session 2002-3 Inequalities in Access to Maternity Services and Ninth report of session 2002-3 Choice in Maternity Services. The Stationery Office, London.

International Confederation of Midwives 1999 International Code of Ethics for Midwives. ICM, London.

Kirkham M 2000 How can we relate? In: Kirkham M (ed), The Midwife–Mother Relationship. Macmillan Press, Hampshire, pp. 227–254.

Kirkham M, Stapleton H, Curtis P, et al. 2002 The inverse care law in midwifery care. British Journal of Midwifery 10(8): 509–519.

Lavender T, Walkinshaw SA, Walton I 1999 A prospective study of women's views of factors contributing to a positive birth experience. Midwifery 15(1): 40–46.

Leap N 2000 The less we do, the more we give. In: Kirkham M (ed), The Midwife–Mother Relationship. Macmillan Press, Hampshire, pp. 1–18.

Levy V 1999a Maintaining equilibrium: a grounded theory study of the processes involved when women make informed choices during pregnancy. Midwifery 15(2): 109–111.

Levy V 1999b Midwives, informed choice and power: part 1. British Journal of Midwifery 7(9): 583–586.

Levy V 1999c Midwives, informed choice and power: part 2. British Journal of Midwifery 7(10): 613–616.

Levy V 1999d Midwives, informed choice and power: part 3. British Journal of Midwifery 7(11): 694–699.

Levy V 1999e Protective steering: a grounded theory study of the processes by which midwives facilitate informed choices during pregnancy. Journal of Advanced Nursing 29(1): 104–112.

NHS Executive 1996 Patient partnership. HMSO, London.

O'Cathain A, Thomas K, Walters SJ, et al. 2002a Women's perceptions of informed choice in maternity care. Midwifery 18(2): 136–144.

O'Cathain A, Walters SJ, Nicholl JP, et al. 2002b Use of evidence base leaflets to promote informed choice in maternity care: randomized controlled trial in everyday practice. British Medical Journal 324(7338): 643–645.

Page LA 2000 Putting science and sensitivity into practice. In: Page LA (ed), The New Midwifery: science and sensitivity in practice. Churchill Livingstone, Edinburgh, pp. 7–44.

Pairman S 2000 Women-centred midwifery: partnerships or professional friendships? In: Kirkham M (ed), The Midwife–Mother Relationship. Macmillan Press, Hampshire, pp. 207–226.

Pairman S, Gulliland K 2003 Developing a midwife-led maternity service: the New Zealand experience. In: Kirkham M (ed), Birth Centres. A social model for maternity care. Books for Midwives, Edinburgh, pp. 223–238.

Phelan JP, Ahn MO, Diaz F, et al. 1989 Twice a caesarean, always a caesarean? Obstetrics and Gynecology 73: 161–165.

Pritchard J 1996 Ethical decision-making and the positive use of codes. In: Frith L (ed), Ethics and Midwifery: issues in contemporary practice. Butterworth-Heinemann, Oxford, pp. 189–204.

Rosen MG, Dickinson JC 1990 Vaginal birth after caesarean: a meta-analysis of indicators for success. Obstetrics and Gynecology 76: 865–869.

Saxell L 2000 Risk: theoretical or actual. In: Page LA (ed), The New Midwifery: science and sensitivity in practice. Churchill Livingstone, Edinburgh, pp. 87–104.

Shapiro MC, Najman JM, Chang A, et al. 1983 Information control and the exercise of power in the obstetrical encounter. Social Science and Medicine 17(3): 139–146.

Stapleton H 1997 Choice in the face of uncertainty. In: Kirkham M, Perkins ER (eds), Reflections on Midwifery. Baillière Tindall, London, pp. 47–69.

Stapleton H 2000 The MIDIRS Informed Choice leaflets in clinical practice. MIDIRS Midwifery Digest 10(3): 388–392.

Stapleton H, Kirkham M, Curtis P, et al. 2002a Silence and time in antenatal care. British Journal of Midwifery 10(6): 393–396.

Stapleton H, Kirkham M, Curtis P, et al. 2002b Framing information in antenatal care. British Journal of Midwifery 10(4): 197–201.

Stapleton H, Kirkham M, Thomas G 2002c Qualitative study of evidence based leaflets in maternity care. British Medical Journal 324(7338): 639–642.

Stapleton H, Kirkham M, Thomas G, et al. 2002d Language use in antenatal consultations. British Journal of Midwifery 10(5): 273–277.

Stapleton H, Kirkham M, Thomas G, et al. 2002e Midwives in the middle: balance and vulnerability. British Journal of Midwifery 10(10): 607–611.

Thomas J, Paranjothy S 2001 The National Sentinel Caesarean Section Audit Report. RCOG, London.

Towle A, Godolphin W 1999 Framework for teaching and learning informed shared decision making. British Medical Journal 319(7212): 766–771.

Towle A, Godolphin W 2001 Education and training of healthcare professionals. In: Edwards A, Elwyn G (eds), Evidence-based Patient Choice: Inevitable or Impossible? Oxford University Press, Oxford, pp. 245–269.

Walsh D, Newburn M 2002 Towards a social model of childbirth: part 1. British Journal of Midwifery 10(8): 476–481.

Wyke S, Hewison J Elton R, et al. 2001 Does general practice involvement in commissioning maternity care make a difference? Journal of Health Services Research and Policy 6: 99–104.

Further Reading

Available websites include:
www.infochoice.org
MIDIRS Informed Choice website. Leaflets for parents and professionals can be downloaded and printed from this site.

www.discern.org.uk
Discern project website. This site gives quality criteria for consumer health information. It includes a very useful proforma of standards to meet when writing or assessing parent information.

www.doh.gov.uk
Department of Health reports can be accessed from this web site.

Chapter 10

The Reflective Practitioner

Kathleen P. Nakielski

INTRODUCTION

Kirkham (1994) identifies reflection as a basis for both professional and personal growth and development. Church and Raynor (2000) believe reflection enables midwives to investigate the factors that guide and shape their practice, and can either assist or hinder working in partnership with women. The Nursing and Midwifery Council (NMC 2004a), as part of the Post Registration Education and Practice (PREP), now requires midwives to provide evidence of lifelong learning, reflect upon practice, and be able to link both theory and practice to improve care. This chapter seeks to clarify the concepts and philosophies of reflection and explore how the reflective process can assist midwives in everyday clinical practice and decision making.

The theoretical concepts of Theories of Action (*espoused theories* and *theories-in-use*), *technical rationality* and Reflection and Action (*reflection-on-action* and *reflection-in-action*) generated by Argyris and Schön (1974) and Schön (1987, 1991) will be explored and set in the context of midwifery practice and decision making.

The Experiential Learning Cycle (Gibbs 1988) will be analysed and its use explored from the perspective of both student and experienced midwife. The advantages and disadvantages of reflective practice to the midwife and the families in her care will also be identified.

Due to the nature of reflection and reflective practice, the personal pronoun will be used within this chapter.

WHAT IS REFLECTION?

Reflection is a normal human activity that is essential to cognitive development and allows personal growth by learning from our experiences, mistakes and successes. Children learn that certain actions bring pain, discomfort and parental disapproval, while others lead to positive regard and approval – thereby learning that there are socially acceptable actions, norms and values. As maturity is reached, it is presumed that this learning process has developed and adults will think of the advantages and disadvantages of each action before they proceed. Boud et al. (1985) discuss the development of this intellectual and emotional activity as a natural event, and note that some adults are more successful than others. Those who learn effectively from experience develop new understandings and appreciations of their environment.

Midwives have traditionally learned from lectures during educational programmes, journals, observation of other midwives' practice and from personal clinical experience. Schön (1991) describes the Reflective Practitioner as someone who learns by reflecting on current experience and applies that learning to future practice.

The term 'experience' is often used as if it is synonymous with learning, but this is not always the case. Dewey (1933) believes that all learning stems from experience, but not all experience results in learning. Midwives do not always recognise the value of daily clinical experience as a learning opportunity (Morgan 2000). Two midwives may have identical experience in clinical practice: one may develop a new understanding of how to be with women, while the other may view it as another working day. The experience is the same; the learning is very different and consequently may result in different decisions being made when caring for women.

Not all learning derived from midwifery practice will be positive. For example, a midwife may change her practice following the birth of an infant with a low Apgar score which was unforeseen and unexplained. The midwife may have monitored the fetal heart during labour intermittently. There were no changes in the fetal heart rate pattern to indicate anything other than normal progress in labour. Rather than re-examining the situation to identify any factors that may have led to this situation, the midwife decided to use continuous electronic fetal monitoring for all women in the future, regardless of the risk assessment, contrary to current best evidence (National Institute for Clinical Excellence [NICE] 2001). Decisions about the care of all future clients are based on an emotional response rather than current evidence, which is unwise. Dewey (1933) would describe this type of learning as dysfunctional. Experiences do not occur in isolation, and the practitioner will respond depending upon their own previous experience.

Atkins and Murphy (1993) have described the literature on reflection as both abstract and complex. This makes concepts difficult to grasp – particularly as authors utilise inconsistent terminology to identify similar key stages in the reflective process. An overview of some of the concepts used in reflection will be identified, and their use in decision making and the improvement of professional practice explored.

THE DEFINITION AND IMPORTANCE OF REFLECTION

In order to understand the concept of reflective practice, certain definitions can be useful. Definitions are numerous within the literature, but those provided by Reid (1993) and Atkins and Murphy (1993) will allow analysis and application to midwifery practice and decision making.

Reid's (1993) definition allows the midwife to analyse the content and evidence base for their practice:

"... *a process of reviewing an experience of practice in order to describe, analyse and evaluate and so inform learning from practice." Reid (1993: 305).*

Midwives have a professional responsibility to act in the best interests of women and their families, and are responsible for both their acts and omissions (Nursing and Midwifery Council [NMC] 2004b). Paul and Heaslip (1995) believe that without critical analysis and vigilance through a process of reflection, clients can be put in danger. Midwives must strive for clinical excellence at all times, otherwise women and their families have to deal with the physical and psychological morbidity and potential mortality of any act or omission. At all times midwives should be able to answer the questions of *who, what, why, where* and *when* surrounding their professional practice. Murphy-Black and Faulkner (1990) state that for midwives to be viewed as independent accountable practitioners they must develop a body of distinct professional knowledge and know *what* they must do and *how* to do it; moreover, they must underpin that knowledge with evidence to answer *why*. It can also be postulated that midwives must also know *who* should make the decisions about the plan of care as lead professional (DoH 1993), and who is best placed to provide that care, whether the midwife, obstetrician, healthcare support worker, lay organisations or family members. The *where* and *when* to provide care should be the joint decision of woman and midwife, and made in the light of the best evidence and fully informed consent. Chapters 2, 4 and 8 of this book explore these concepts further.

All healthcare professionals are required to base their decisions and individual practice within a framework of evidence-based knowledge (DoH 1993, 1997, 1998, NHS Executive 2000, NMC 2004b). Murphy-Black and Faulkner (1990) identify that what is ideal practice today may be discarded tomorrow as research demonstrates its flaws. It is no longer acceptable for any midwife still to use the knowledge gained at the point of registration throughout their career without constant re-evaluation (NMC 2004b). Educational programmes encourage the acquisition of the skills necessary to search and evaluate the literature to ensure that decisions and practice are evidence-based (NMC 2004c). A review of this process can be found in Chapter 4.

Atkins and Murphy (1993: 1191) move on from Reid's (1993) definition stating:

". . . reflection . . . must involve the self and must lead to a changed perspective. It is these crucial aspects which distinguish reflection from analysis."

The reflective process requires the examination of self and for the midwife to examine their beliefs, values and attitudes. Boyd and Fales (1983) identify that the reflective process is triggered by a personal sense of discomfort. Mezirow (1981) describes the involvement of self as 'perspective transformation' – a process whereby one becomes critically aware of how customary ways of thinking and acting limit or distort understanding of one's self or others. This perspective transformation can be the result of a sudden insight, possibly as the result of a critical incident, into the whole structure of one's assumptions. Or it may occur over a period of time due to a growing awareness of a precise notion that may be modified slowly.

THE ROLE OF INTUITION

Church and Raynor (2000) acknowledge that over recent years the emphasis on academic and experimentally derived knowledge has vastly increased, and that there is the potential for practice and experience to become devalued. An experienced practitioner may utilise knowledge of biology, physiology, behavioural sciences and the latest research evidence to underpin their practice, and is able to articulate their use of this knowledge quite clearly. However, they may find it difficult to quantify the influence that years of clinical experience and intuition (see Chapter 7) has had on their decisions and practice. However, they will be able to identify its use by recounting occasions when lives were saved by making an intuitive decision. Burnard (1989) suggests that intuition by its nature cannot be empirically defined, but that this 'sixth sense' is a very important way of knowing how to care and must be listened to and explored thorough reflective writing.

Benner's (1984) phenomenological work explores the development of nurses from novice to expert practitioners, and the role that intuition has in this transition. A novice has no experience of the clinical situation – they need to gain experience of tasks and procedures, and have been taught context-free rules to guide their actions. The novice can perform simple tasks and discuss the basic principles that underpin practice. However, as the level of expertise increases, so does the use of intuition in clinical decision making. Experts are those who are skilled in tasks and procedures. Their intuitive nursing action has become so refined that they are unable to define the cognitive process they use to make their decisions. Reflection can be used by the novice to link theory and practice and to set goals for future learning. It can also be used by the expert to ensure that their practice is evidence-based and to attempt to articulate their use of experience and intuition in their decision making.

THEORIES OF ACTION

Argyris and Schön (1974) and Schön (1987, 1991) identified two theories of action which inform individual patterns of interpersonal behaviour, espoused theories and theories-in-use.

ESPOUSED THEORIES

Espoused theories are theories which practitioners say that they use in everyday practice and are readily communicated to others, while theories-in-use are those actually used in everyday practice. Greenwood (1993) believes that espoused theory is theory disseminated by educational institutions and from literature as 'midwifery theory'. Midwifery espoused theory would encompass the beliefs that every woman is a unique autonomous individual (see Chapters 1 and 9) who is able to make informed decisions about her care, that each woman should be actively involved in her individualised care, and that birth is a prospectively normal process.

THEORIES-IN-USE

Theories-in-use are learned through the real world of clinical experience, and may have developed unconsciously. These beliefs may be congruent with espoused theory and allow effective decision making and care provision. Incongruent theories-in-use may focus on a condition or complication rather than the woman as a whole; they may centre on getting through the workload rather than meeting individual needs, and may only see birth as normal in retrospect. Conflict arises if the espoused and theories-in-use differ or are incompatible, and this may explain why midwives may not always practice what they preach and are unaware that this is the case. Without reflection, Argyris and Schön (1974) believe that practitioners will remain unaware of tacit (unspoken) theories-in-use and its effects on decision-making. Schön (1987) believes that theories-in-use are generally used in difficult or stressful situations. Kirkham (1997) echoed that at times of stress, discomfort in midwifery practice is ignored and suppressed until triggered by words from a colleague or client.

TECHNICAL RATIONALITY

Schön (1991) used the term technical rationality to describe the 'applied science' view of professional practice. Professionals attempt to solve problems through the application of scientific theory and techniques using a systematic problem-solving approach taught during their educational programmes. Greenwood (1993) identifies that difficulties occur with the application of a technical rationality approach because problems may not have been identified, or that the end point is not clear or readily agreed upon. Schön (1987) sees research-based theory as solving unimportant and easy-to-solve problems on the 'high ground', while those of greatest human concern are confusing problems which defy technical solutions and reside in the swampy lowland. Midwifery practice frequently provides situations where the problems are not clearly defined but are of greatest human concern. The artistry of professional practice is the ability to select an appropriate frame to structure the problem. A frame being a strategy used by a professional to define the problem, which carries a tacit response to that situation (Schön 1991). The decisions made in practice are based on an individual practitioner's tacit frames. Schön (1991) views reflection as the link between academic knowledge and science and practical competence and professional artistry.

REFLECTION AND ACTION

Schön (1987, 1991) further theorises that there are two rudiments of reflective practice – reflection-on-action and reflection-in-action.

REFLECTION-ON-ACTION

Reflection-on-action is described is a 'cognitive post-mortem' (Greenwood 1993), where the practitioner explores the situation in light of the outcomes. This may be the more frequently used method of reflection in midwifery practice (Tiran 2003), as reflection is more likely to occur following the recognition of uncomfortable feelings (Boyd and Fales 1983). Unexpected outcomes following decisions and actions in midwifery may trigger this retrospective analysis of individual practice. Reflection-on-action allows the midwife to speculate on alternative methods, knowledge or decisions that would have been helpful. Student midwives may find reflection-on-action to be a useful approach that contributes to continuing development of skills, knowledge and setting goals for future practice.

REFLECTION-IN-ACTION

Reflection-in-action (Schön 1987, 1991) occurs while practising. The practitioner selects and re-mixes responses from previous experiences when deciding how to solve a problem in practice and utilising their tacit frames. Reflection-in-action is thought to promote the skilled and flexible response of the expert practitioner (Benner 1984). Greenwood (1998) believes that the Argyris and Schön (1974) and Schön (1987, 1991) theories of reflection are defective because they omit the concept of reflection-before-action. It is always wise for midwives to think before they act.

DIFFICULTIES WITH LEARNING FROM PRACTICE

Some individuals choose not to reflect or learn in either their personal lives or professional practice. In Box 10.1, Jarvis (1995) categorises those individuals who do not learn from experience as 'non-learning', and describes three categories of non-learner.

Box 10.1   Categories of Non-Learner

1. *Presumption*: those whose previous experiences have provided sufficient learning and that the repetition of previous responses will suffice.
2. *Non-consideration*: they are too busy to think about learning from a situation, or they fear the outcome of the thought process.
3. *Rejection*: they think about the possibility of learning from experience, but feel they will not have their opinions or attitudes changed by the world.

Reference: Jarvis P 1995 Adult and Continuing Education. Theory and Practice. 2nd edition. Routledge, London, pp. 71–72.

Non-learners potentially make decisions based on outdated information, and do not learn from women or the current evidence. Main (1985) identifies that long-established patterns of behaviour are enduring and difficult to change. Habitual practice has a reassuring element for the midwife; performance is constant and self-sustaining. When changing practice, performance will be less effective, and Main (1985) terms this change as 'conscious incompetence'. The midwife will find this change in performance disconcerting, and may revert to habitual practice if support and reassurance to maintain the improved level of performance is not available. The fear of perceived change in competence may prevent midwives from reflecting and learning from their practice.

Jarvis and Gibson (1997) believe that to prevent non-learning, midwives need to act as reflective role models and support junior colleagues. There is also a need for the National Health Service (NHS) to acknowledge that learning and reflecting periods are essential, and these should be built into the midwives' role and job description. However, Main (1985) cautions against an habitual approach to learning because this prevents discovery of theories-in-use. The supervisor of midwives has a role in supporting the reflection on practice (Caldwell 1996), and midwives may choose to support each other in this process through reflective practice groups (Hansom and Butler 2003).

REFLECTIVE SKILLS AND MODELS OF REFLECTION

Reflection is essential for professional practice, and should be undertaken in a structured way. Adults develop personal paradigms to structure reflection in everyday life. Undertaking Activity 10.1 should help to clarify your personal construct.

During Activity 10.1, many of the skills required to be reflective may have been identified (Atkins and Murphy 1993), and these are highlighted in Box 10.2. The subject may have been chosen because of an uncomfortable

---

✎ Activity 10.1

Think of a recent situation in your personal life that you discussed with a friend or family member. Try to think of the process

- What where the key features of the discussion?
- What have you learned, and why?
- Has the situation changed your views?
- What would you do if it happened again?
- Has this situation been recounted to others? If so has it changed with time?

---

feeling that arose from the incident. This self-awareness is consistent with Boyd and Fales' (1983) theory of why reflection occurs. The descriptive phase is necessary so that the listener can understand the uncomfortable feeling that the situation had stimulated. Depending upon the context of the situation, the description may not have been totally accurate. Newell (1992) identifies that memory of an incident may change over time. Inaccuracies may occur because of the degradation of the memory. Stress and anxiety at the time of the incident may have led to a misinterpretation of the situation, and therefore faulty memory. The description of the incident may change each time it is recounted to place the teller in the most favourable light. This is of particular importance if the description damages the teller's concept of self and self-esteem. Critical analysis requires the midwife to scrutinise the

---

Box 10.2 The Skills Required to be Reflective

- Self-awareness
- Description
- Critical analysis
- Synthesis
- Evaluation

Source: Atkins S, Murphy K 1993 Reflection: a review of the literature. Journal of Advanced Nursing 18: 1190.

components of the situation by isolating existing knowledge, testing assumptions (particularly the identification of espoused theories and theories-in-use) and to discover alternatives. Synthesis is the integration of new and previous knowledge. Stephenson (1985) goes on to describe synthesis as contemplating all possible results from a course of action before using this information to make a decision and solve a clinical problem. Midwives use this ability to greatest effect when they reflect-in-action. Evaluation allows the midwife to take a judgement on the value of the experience.

For reflection to take place in a structured, constructive and effective way, the use of a model of reflection is essential. The model must meet both professional needs and personal preference. It must allow the review of feeling, ideas and concepts that underpin practice, and encourage the practitioner to locate/relocate their decisions and practice in current research and literature. The frequency of use is of paramount importance in the choice of a model of reflection. The more user-friendly the model, the more frequent it will be used.

There are a vast number of reflective models available in the literature, and time should be taken to make the correct choice based on personal preference. Those models by Johns (2000: 47), Atkins and Murphy (1993: 1191), Boud et al. (1985: 36) and Reid's (2000: 83) modification of Gibbs (1988) model are worth considering, but the construction of a personal model is not inappropriate.

The Experiential Learning Cycle was first identified by Gibbs (1988) to help students clarify the learning experience. Dewey (1933) believes that learning is not cyclical, but spiral, with each experience creating the potential to move to the next experience and continue the learning process. Figure 10.1 modifies the Experiential Learning Cycle to reflect the spiral nature of reflective practice. Gibbs (1988) originally described a seven-point cyclical model, but this has been modified to combine conclusions that are general and specific to one point (point 5) on the model (Figure 10.1 and Table 10.1). It is important to remember that the descriptive section should be just that – making judgements

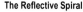

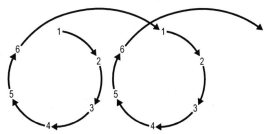

Number on the spiral relates to phases 1 to 6 of Table 10.1

Figure 10.1 The Reflective Spiral (Adapted from Dewey J [1933] How We Think. D C Health, Boston.)

and drawing conclusions should occur later. Clear descriptions will assist in the identification of issues to be analysed at a later point in the model. Reactions and feelings should also be recorded without analysis – by analysing at this stage, it would be difficult to become aware of ritualistic practice and theories-in-use.

KEEPING A REFLECTIVE JOURNAL

As can be seen from the works of Atkins and Murphy (1993) and Gibbs (1988), the activity of description is essential for reflection to take place. The reflective writing represents a convenient way to commence this activity. The terminology differs in the literature, describing this written record as a log, a diary, or a journal (Stuart 1997) to a portfolio (McMullan et al. 2003). Stuart (1997) identifies that keeping a reflective journal requires a clear understanding of the concept of reflection and the possession of reflective skills (Atkins and Murphy 1993).

Student midwives are encouraged to keep reflective journals to assist them in producing reflective portfolios as part of their assessment of competence. McMullan et al. (2003) recognise that students use portfolios and the reflective process to revalidate and record strengths, skills and knowledge. A portfolio also promotes the link of theory to practice, problem-solving skills, self-awareness and critical thinking. It can also be presumed that portfolios prepare students for lifelong learning and continued reflective practice.

Table 10.1   The Experiential Learning Cycle

Phase	Title of Phase	Questions
1	Description	What happened?
2	Feelings	What were your reactions and feelings?
3	Evaluation	What was good and bad about the experience?
4	Analysis	What sense can you make of the situation?
		What was really going on?
		Were different people's experiences similar or different in important ways?
5	Conclusion (general)	What can be concluded, in a general sense, from these experiences and the analysis you have undertaken?
	Conclusion (specific)	What can be concluded about your own specific, unique, personal situation or way of working?
6	Personal action plan	What are you going to do differently in this type of situation next time?
		What steps are you going to take on the basis of what you have learnt?

Source: Modified from Gibbs G 1988 Learning by Doing: a Guide to Teaching and Learning Methods. Further Education Unit Oxford Polytechnic, Oxford, p. 46.

It is essential that all entries in a reflective journal have no identifying information in order to maintain the confidentiality and anonymity of women, families (NMC 2004b), professionals and locations. Hargreaves (1997) questions the use of a written record to detail care and undertake reflection without the woman's knowledge and informed consent.

Entries are made in response to a critical incident. The term 'critical' refers to incidents which are critical to the midwife's learning but are not life-threatening. Entries must be made frequently in order to develop reflective skills and relocate practice decisions in the literature.

REFLECTION ON A CRITICAL INCIDENT

The activity of reflection will be explored by reviewing entries in the reflective journals of a student midwife and an experienced community midwife (Practical examples 10.1 and 10.2, respectively) and demonstrate how Gibbs (1988) Experiential Learning Cycle (Table 10.1) was used differently, but with the same result.

Practical Example 10.1

Lisa is a student midwife entering her second year of training, and is currently undertaking community midwifery experience. This reflective piece is recorded as part of the reflective journal, which demonstrates her evidence of learning in clinical practice. The entry had been made two days after the event.

1. Description
I attended my first home birth with my community midwife Mike. I had met Sandra and Dave twice over the last 3 weeks as we helped them to prepare for their home birth. Sandra was a primigravida, and she had made the decision to give birth at home. Mike had contacted me at 05:00 and informed me that Sandra was in labour and happy for me to attend.

Sandra's labour had started at around midnight. By 06:00, her contractions were coming every 3 minutes and she was relaxing in the bath. I assisted Mike in taking the observations and recording them on the partogram; everything was progressing normally. Sandra never asked for analgesia throughout the labour. Baby Susan was born at 09:15 with Apgars of 9 at 1 minute and 9 at 10 minutes; she weighed

3.825 kg. The placenta and membranes were delivered by maternal effort at 10:00. Sandra had a small labial graze and the blood loss was estimated at 100 ml.

2. Feelings

I was amazed how relaxed Sandra had been. I had never seen a primigravida so in control of the situation, or so in tune with her body. It was a powerful experience.

I felt confused – how can a primigravida cope without any analgesia?

I was concerned about the third stage of labour. It appeared as it was just left to happen. I realised I know nothing about how to manage this situation, and that scares me.

3. Evaluation

It was fantastic! It was a privilege to be there. Sandra was calm and in charge of the situation. She decided when to get in and out of the bath, where to walk, and what to eat and drink. I am aware I need to develop the skills to encourage other women to do this.
This situation has made me realise that my knowledge needs to be increased in these areas.

4. Analysis

I realised that I need to review my knowledge of physiology and promoting normality. I reviewed the following texts: Robertson (2000), Wagner (1994) and Balaskas (1991). I am aware of the effects of adrenaline on endorphins and oxytocin production and slowing labour. I must do everything within my power to reduce stress and promote women's control over the labour environment. It had deepened my knowledge of mobility and positions in labour.

I commenced by re-reading McDonald's (2003) chapter on the physiology and management of the third stage. I still had some unanswered questions, so I progressed to review Inch's (1985) work on the physiological management of the third stage and Rogers et al.'s (1998) Hinchingbrooke third stage trial.

5. Conclusion

There was nothing else I could have done but experience this wonderful birth. I have now witnessed a totally physiological birth, and have seen that it is possible for a primigravida to give birth at home.

6. Action plan

I am so much more aware and prepared for my role in the helping to promote normality in labour. I have a better understanding and can use the literature and research to offer informed choice. I am ready for my next birth!

✓ Practical Example 10.2

Sally is a community midwife with 20 years' experience. She had been called to the Labour Ward at a busy time to help. This is an extract from her reflective journal written the day after the critical incident.

I arrived on the labour ward at 09:15. It was very busy, but I felt confident in the environment thanks to my one shift per month in the unit. There were five women in labour, and an emergency Caesarean section in progress with five midwives on duty. Katie had just arrived, apparently in labour.

09:20: I was asked to admit Katie. This was Katie's second pregnancy; it had been a healthy pregnancy now at term+2. Katie's previous pregnancy had been induced at term+10, but had been normal. She had required a ventouse extraction for prolonged second stage. Her labour had been 16 hours long, with an epidural for pain relief.

Simon, Katie's partner was present. Contractions started at 04:30 and were now coming 3 in 10 moderate and lasting 40 seconds. The membranes where intact and the fetal heart was heard strongly as 138 bpm with the pinard's stethoscope. I decided that intermittent auscultation of the fetal heart was appropriate as I had confirmed she was low risk (NICE 2001). I reviewed the birth plan and talked it through with the couple. Katie was very keen to have another epidural. I explained that the anaesthetist was busy in theatre and it would be some time before she would be available.

We discussed Katie's options between contractions, and she appeared surprised to hear the advantages and disadvantages of her analgesia options. We discussed the issues surrounding epidural analgesia, and how Katie perceived its effects in the last labour. With this information Katie decided that she would like to try a labour without pharmacological analgesia.

10:15: During this discussion Katie had been mobile and contractions had now become 4 in 10 and a little stronger. I auscultated the fetal heart every 15 minutes, and had commenced the partogram. I was pleased to find a new birth ball in the room; the balls had just arrived in the unit. I had read the article by Shallow (2003) on their use, so I actively encouraged Katie to try the birthing ball. She appeared surprised just how comfortable it was and allowed her to rest a little.

10:30: The labour ward coordinator knocked on the door and asked for an update on the situation. I reported that Katie was progressing well and at low risk. It was requested that I undertake a vaginal examination to confirm established labour. I was unable to debate my objections at length because of Katie requiring my support.

10:45: I discussed the option of undertaking a vaginal examination with Katie. She was surprised I had not requested to do so earlier. During the examination I confirmed that Katie's cervix was 8 cm dilated. I informed Katie of the findings, and then the labour ward coordinator.

11:10: Katie became very distressed and was obviously in transition. She requested an epidural. Simon also appeared very distressed and asked me to do something. I reminded them that we had discussed earlier that this may happen at this point. Katie decided to use Entonox.

11:15: There was a spontaneous rupture of membranes, the liquor was clear, and the fetal heart rate was 120 bpm. Katie commenced spontaneous pushing.

11:31: Katie gave birth to a daughter, who was born in good condition and went straight to the breast.

11:46: The placenta and membranes arrived following an expectant management.

Katie and Simon were elated, and thanked me for my help and support in the birth of their daughter. I feel mixed emotions at this birth. I feel elated that I had encouraged Katie to experience the birth process with minimal analgesia and had avoided the use of an epidural, but I feel angry that I had been pressurised into undertaking a vaginal examination. I knew she was in normal established labour, and I did not need to do a vaginal examination to see that. I felt confident that things where going well and I was responsible and was prepared to stand by my decisions.

Katie had not anticipated a 'natural birth' and had already decided upon an epidural prior to labour. She had not read nor been informed of her options, and had relied on her previous experience of labour. I had been so confident that she was able to labour without medication and clearly conveyed that confidence.

I was so shocked that I was required to undertake a vaginal examination. I had almost forgotten that I was in the hospital environment. I was practising, as I would have done in Katie's home being observant but not intrusive, taking responsibility and acting as an autonomous accountable practitioner. I had forgotten the need to mention everything about labour when in the hospital environment. I had moved from prospectively to retrospectively normal.

Having thought about this, have I become obsessed by keeping things normal? Could I have offered Katie pain relief rather than trying out the birth ball? Had I denied her the analgesia she had anticipated in order to promote my beliefs and use the ball? Had I over-ridden her wishes? I don't believe so. Katie had remained in control throughout. I had offered analgesia at transition because I knew both she and Simon were scared and needed the confidence that it would give. They thanked me for my care. Would they have done that if I had not helped?

Why am I so angry about undertaking a vaginal examination? Katie had consented and had expected this assessment? I know that there is no research basis for the frequency and timing of vaginal examinations in labour (Devane 1996). Stuart (2003) agrees with me that other methods of assessing progress in labour such as the descent of the fetal head are just as valid. I think I am angry with myself for not standing up for my beliefs. Also that some midwives and obstetricians have become obsessed by making decisions and managing labour on vaginal examinations alone (Walsh 2000). The birthing ball had helped in the way I had expected (Shallow 2003).

I plan to contact Katie and Simon to check that they were happy with the care they received. I don't believe I would care for Katie differently, except for not undertaking the vaginal examination. I would definitely encourage use of the birthing ball again.

The reflective writing in Practical Example 10.1 is now compared and contrasted with Practical Example 10.2.

Lisa (the student midwife) and Sally (the community midwife) had approached the reflective process differently, but both are equally valid and demonstrate the use of reflective skills. As an inexperienced reflector, Lisa chose the security headings to ensure she had followed the process. Sally was confident and had the experience to work intuitively.

Lisa used the process to identify uncomfortable feelings about her level of knowledge and to address this deficiency through reading; hence, she is better prepared for the next time she is exposed to this situation. Sally used the process to locate her practice in the literature and ensure that the decisions she made were based on the best evidence. The uncomfortable feelings generated questions which exposed Sally's espoused theories and theories-in-use and the influence these have on her decision-making skills. Kirkham (1997) recommends that women are involved in our reflective processes to be seen as others see us, and to explore the influence that our decisions have on the recipients.

Both Lisa and Sally are aware of the autonomy of the woman and its influence on their practice. Sally also has a well-developed sense of her professional accountability and role as advocate. She is doubting her ability to empower women and maintain their autonomy, but this awareness should help her to address the issues.

Lisa primarily used reflection-on-action to reduce the theory practice gap (McMullan et al. 2003). This is appropriate for a student at this point because she has insufficient experience and knowledge to reflect-in-action. Sally is using experience, knowledge and intuition to reflect-in-action.

ADVANTAGES AND LIMITATIONS OF REFLECTION

Self-examination during reflection can be both frightening and exciting. This fear may be a barrier to the practice of reflection, stemming from an unwillingness to explore the difference between espoused theories and theories-in-use and expose deficiency in personal practice. The midwife may feel anxiety or worse, and have no one they feel they can turn to for advice and support. The importance of supervision and support within an atmosphere of trust and confidentiality must be stressed (Fish et al. 1991, Paterson 1995, Hansom and Butler 2003), especially if the reflection identifies that they put a client at risk by their action or omission (NMC 2004b).

Kirkham (1997) identifies that the midwife's professional and personal defence mechanisms may make it difficult to view their practice as colleagues and clients would do. Midwives must be aware that the effects of stress and anxiety at the time of incidents will affect recall and willingness to record the incident reflectively (Newell 1992). Repression of some of the more distressing elements of an incident may occur. Midwives may refuse to confront any decisions or practice that they find distasteful or detrimental to their concept of self and professional identity. Unless this is addressed, learning will not take place and care and decision-making abilities will not improve.

McMullan et al. (2003) identified that students need to feel confident that the content of their reflective portfolio will be confidential, otherwise self-censorship of the content will occur and reduce its impact. Midwives also find difficulty in writing reflectively because it requires the use of the personal pronoun and the activities of critical analysis and synthesis. This will lead to work which is either totally descriptive and without linkage to theory, or is academic without the use of self. Reflection should be a marriage of both, but this skill takes time to develop.

Dysfunctional learning must be avoided at all costs. It is particularly important that midwives are given support and guidance through midwifery supervision to prevent this (Duerden 2003). The modern face of midwifery supervision, in being distinct from midwifery management, should help to prevent the dysfunctional learning which may previously have led to defensive practice that encouraged the philosophy of normal in retrospect. Midwifery supervision can also be used to challenge the attitudes of non-learners (Jarvis 1995), and encourage midwives to engage in reviewing their professional performance by offering insight and support with their individual difficulties.

The use of reflection to add insight into practice appears sound, but no rigorous research studies have been conducted on the use of reflection in midwifery to confirm this (Kirkham 1997, Fitzgerald 1994). The development of reflective skills is not always easy, but it can be rewarding and has positive benefits on the midwife's ability to make decisions.

The midwife is able to constantly review individual practice to ensure that it is woman-centred and evidence-based.

CONCLUSION

This chapter has explored the concept of reflective practice, and demonstrates how reflection is essential for effective clinical practice and decision making. The reflective journal entries demonstrate that the use of reflective skills and models are essential for lifelong learning and evidence-based, woman-centred decision making. The text can be used to assist both qualified and student midwives to develop reflective skills.

KEY POINTS FOR BEST PRACTICE

- Reflection is essential for modern midwifery practice. Midwives must be able to answer the *who*, *what*, *why*, *where* and *when* which underpins all aspects of their individual practice.

- The midwife must closely examine the beliefs, values and attitudes that are used and expressed in their practice. Midwives must practise (theories-in-use) what they preach (espoused theories).

- Reflection allows midwives to explore the art (intuition) and science (evidence base) which is the foundation of practice.

- Reflective models assist the midwife to clarify the concepts that support practice and encourages the location/relocation of their practice and decisions in current literature and research.

- A reflective model should be chosen to encourage the frequency of use. Constant reflection–on–action will encourage the development of the skill of reflection–in–action.

- Women deserve care provided by skilled reflective practitioners.

References

Argyris C, Schön DA 1974 Theory in Practice. Jossey-Bass, San Francisco.

Atkins S, Murphy K 1993 Reflection: a review of the literature. Journal of Advanced Nursing 18: 1188–1192.

Balaskas J 1991 New Active Birth. A Concise Guide to Natural Childbirth. Thorsons, London.

Benner P 1984 From Novice to Expert: Excellence and Power in Clinical Nursing Practice. Addison-Wesley Publishing Company, California.

Boud D, Keogh R, Walker D 1985 Promoting Reflection in Learning: a Model. In: Boud D, Keogh R, Walker D (eds), Reflection: Turning Experience into Learning. Kogan Page, London, pp. 18–40.

Boyd EM, Fales AW 1983 Reflective learning – key to learning from experience. Journal of Humanistic Psychology 23: 99–117.

Burnard P 1989 The 'sixth sense'. Nursing Times 85(50): 52–53.

Caldwell K 1996 Care for the carers in Exeter. In: Kirkham M (ed), Supervision of Midwives. Books for Midwives, Hale, pp. 84–89.

Church P, Raynor MD 2000 Reflection and articulating intuition. In: Fraser D (ed), Professional Studies for Midwifery Practice. Churchill Livingstone, London.

Department of Health 1993 Changing Childbirth. Report of the Expert Maternity Group. HMSO, London, pp. 23–43.

Department of Health 1997 The new NHS: modern, dependable. HMSO, London.

Department of Health 1998 A first Class Service: quality in the NHS. HMSO, London.

Dewey J 1933 How we think. D C Health, Boston.

Devane D 1996 Sexuality and Midwifery. British Journal of Midwifery 4(8): 413–416.

Duerden J 2003 Supervision of Midwives and Clinical Governance. In: Fraser DM, Cooper MA (eds), Myles Textbook for Midwives. Churchill Livingstone, Edinburgh, pp. 959–973.

Fish D, Twinn S, Purr B 1991 Promoting Reflection: Improving the supervision of practice in Health Visiting and initial teacher training. West London Institute of Higher Education, London.

Fitzgerald M 1994 Theories of reflection for learning. In: Palmer A, Burns S, Bulman C (eds), Reflective Practice in Nursing. The Growth of the Professional Practitioner. Blackwell Scientific Publications, London, pp. 63–84.

Gibbs G 1988 Learning by Doing: a Guide to Teaching and Learning Methods. Further Education Unit Oxford Polytechnic (now Oxford Brooks University), Oxford.

Greenwood J 1993 Reflective practice: a critique of the work of Argyris and Schön. Journal of Advanced Nursing 18: 1183–1187.

Greenwood J 1998 The role of reflection in single and double loop learning. Journal of Advanced Nursing 27(5): 1048–1053.

Hansom J, Butler M 2003 Sharing reflections in midwifery practice. British Journal of Midwifery 11(1): 34–37.

Hargreaves J 1997 Using patients: exploring the ethical dimension of reflective practice in nurse education. Journal of Advanced Nursing 25(2): 223–228.

Inch S 1985 Management of the third stage of labour – another cascade of intervention. Midwifery 1: 114–122.

Jarvis P 1992 Reflective practice and nursing. Nurse Education Today 12: 174–181.

Jarvis P 1995 Adult and Continuing Education. Theory and Practice, 2nd edition. Routledge, London, pp. 71–72.

Jarvis P, Gibson S 1997 The Teacher Practitioner and Mentor in Nursing, Midwifery, Health Visiting and Social Services, 2nd edition. Stanley Thornes Ltd, Cheltenham.

Johns C 2000 Becoming a Reflective Practitioner. Blackwell Science, London.

Kirkham M 1994 Using research skills in midwifery practice. British Journal of Midwifery 2(8): 390–392.

Kirkham M 1997 Reflection in midwifery: professional narcissism or seeing with women? British Journal of Midwifery 5(5): 259–262.

Main A 1985 Reflection and the development of Learning skills. In: Boud D, Keogh R, Walker D (eds), Reflection: Turning Experience into Learning. Kogan Page, London, pp. 91–99

McDonald S 2003 Physiology and Management of the Third Stage of Labour. In: Fraser DM, Cooper MA (eds), Myles Textbook for Midwives. Churchill Livingstone, Edinburgh, pp. 507–530.

McMullan M, Endacott R, Gray MA, Jasper M, Miller C, Scholes J, Webb C 2003 Portfolios and assessment of competence: a review of the literature. Journal of Advanced Nursing 41(3): 283–294.

Mezirow J 1981 A critical theory of adult learning and education. Adult Education 32(1): 3–24.

Morgan R 2000 Lifelong learning. In: Fraser D (ed), Professional Studies for Midwifery Practice. Churchill Livingstone, London, pp. 199–124.

Murphy-Black T, Faulkner A 1990 Midwifery. Excellence in Nursing the Research Route. Scutari Press, London.

National Institute for Clinical Excellence (NICE) 2001 The use of electronic fetal monitoring. The use and interpretation of cardiotocography in intrapartum fetal surveillance. NICE, London.

Newell R 1992 Anxiety, accuracy and reflection: the limits of professional development.

Journal of Advanced Nursing 17: 1326–1333.

NHS Executive 2000 The NHS Plan. A Plan for Investment, a Plan for Reform. HMSO, London.

Nursing and Midwifery Council 2004a The PREP Handbook. NMC, London.

Nursing and Midwifery Council 2004b Code of Professional Conduct: standards for conduct, performance and ethics. NMC, London.

Nursing and Midwifery Council 2004c Standards of Proficiency for Pre-Registration Midwifery Education. NMC, London.

Paterson B 1995 Developing and maintaining reflection in clinical journals. Nurse Education Today 15: 221–220.

Paul RW, Heaslip P 1995 Critical thinking and intuitive nursing practice. Journal of Advanced Nursing 22: 40–47.

Reid B 1993 'But we're doing it already!' Exploring a response to the concept of

Reflective Practice in order to improve its facilitation. Nurse Education Today 13: 305–309.

Reid B 2000 The role of the mentor to aid reflective practice. In: Burns S, Bulman C (eds), Reflective Practice in Nursing. The Growth of the Professional Practitioner, 2nd edition. Blackwell Scientific Publications, London, pp. 79–105.

Robertson A 2000 Tell me about the pain. The Practising Midwife 3(7): 46–47.

Rogers J, Wood J, McClandish R, Ayres S, Truedale A, Elbourne D 1998 Active verses expectant management of the third stage of labour: the Hinchingbrooke randomised controlled trial. The Lancet 351: 693–699.

Schön DA 1987 Educating the Reflective Practitioner. Jossey-Bass, San Francisco.

Schön DA 1991 The Reflective Practitioner: how professionals think in action. Jossey-Bass, San Francisco.

Shallow H 2003 My rolling

programme. The birth ball: ten years experience of using the physiotherapy ball for labouring women. MIDIRS Midwifery Digest 13(1): 28–30.

Stephenson PM 1985 Content of academic essays. Nurse Education Today 5: 81–87.

Stuart CC 1997 Reflective journals as a teacher/learning strategy: a literature review. British Journal of Midwifery 5(7): 434–438.

Stuart CC 2003 Invasive actions in labour. Where have the 'old tricks' gone? In: Wickham S (ed), Midwifery Best Practice. Books for Midwives, Edinburgh, pp. 79–82.

Tiran D 2003 Baillière's Midwives' Dictionary. Baillière Tindall, Edinburgh.

Walsh D 2000 Part Three: Assessing women's progress in labour. British Journal of Midwifery 8(7): 449–457.

Wagner M 1994 Pursuing the birth machine. The Search for Appropriate Birth Technology. ACE Graphics Camperdown, Australia.

Further Reading

Burns S, Bulman C (eds) 2000 Reflective Practice in Nursing. The Growth of the Professional Practitioner, 2nd edition. Blackwell Scientific Publications, London.
A key text which explores many aspects of professional reflective practice.

Carr W, Kemmis S 1986 Becoming Critical. Education, knowledge and action research. The Falmer Press, London.
Explores the concept of reflective practice.

James CR, Clark BA 1994 Reflective practice in nursing: issues and implications for nurse education. Nurse Education Today 14: 82–90.
Explores the issues surrounding the use of reflective journals in professional education

Johns C, Freshwater D 1998 Transforming Nursing Through Reflective Practice. Blackwell Science, Oxford.

Explores the development of reflective practice in nursing.

Kirkham MJ, Perkins ER (eds) 1997 Reflections on Midwifery. Baillière Tindall, London.
Explores the development and use of reflective practice in midwifery.

Nursing and Midwifery Council 2002 Employers and PREP. Information for employers of registered nurses and midwives about post-registration education and practice. NMC, London. Originally printed by the United Kingdom Central Council For Nursing, Midwifery & Health Visiting in 2000.
Provides guidance for employers that post-registration education and practice (PREP) is essential for maintenance of registration and how they can support and encourage practitioners to maintain continued professional development (CPD).

Steele R 1998 Reflection as a way of gathering evidence for your portfolio. RCM Journal (mid-month supplement) May, pp. 4–5.
Provides information to assist the midwife in constructing their evidence of the profession learning required for re-registration.

Wellard SJ, Bethune E 1996 Reflective journal writing in nurse education: whose interests does it serve? Journal of Advanced Nursing 24: 1077–1082.
Explores the issues surrounding the use of reflective journals in professional education.

Watson SJ 1991 An analysis of the concept of experience. Journal of Advanced Nursing 16: 1117–1121.
Explores the literature on the concept of experience.

Chapter **11**

Supporting Decision Making through Supervision

Jean M. Duerden

CHAPTER CONTENTS

INTRODUCTION

Supervision is the ideal paradigm when making an effective clinical or ethical decision. Bound in statute initially by the Midwives Act (House of Commons 1902) and currently by the Nurses, Midwives and Health Visitors' Act (House of Commons 1997), the statutory supervision of midwives provides clear direction as to the most appropriate decision in a given midwifery situation. The grounded principles of supervision assist the decision-maker but, probably of even greater importance, is the ability to use the supervisor of midwives as a sounding board. When midwives were interviewed during audits of supervision of midwives in 1994 (Duerden 1995) and in 1996 (Stapleton et al. 1998), time and again they spoke of using their supervisors in this way. In any of life's decisions, to share the decision-making process or bounce ideas off another person will always enhance, and often ease, the process. This chapter explores the role of the supervisor in facilitating decision making. Practice examples are included as illustrations.

THE ROLE OF THE SUPERVISOR

The role of the supervisor of midwives is to protect the public from sub-optimal care or professional misconduct by a midwife (NMC, 2004b). In essence, however, from the midwives' point of view (Duerden 2000), the role is principally about supporting midwives. Where midwives receive such support and feel empowered by their supervisors they, in turn, empower the women they care for (Stapleton et al. 1998).

The responsibilities of a supervisor of midwives are wide and various, from the receipt of notifications of intention to practise as a midwife from every midwife on the supervisor's case load, to reporting serious cases involving professional misconduct where the Nursing and Midwifery Council (NMC) rules, standards and codes have been contravened. The latter is rarely necessary, as few midwives are guilty of professional misconduct. This does not mean, however, that midwives never practise sub-optimally, either knowingly or unwittingly, but where there is sub-optimal practice, supervisors of midwives can assist midwives in recognising that their practice is below standard and then support them in changing that practice. The close relationship that supervisors have with midwives should mean that they are aware of midwives' practice and, if there are gaps in knowledge or experience, a supervisor should be able to facilitate a midwife in filling these gaps. An example of this is shown in Box 11.1.

The English National Board (ENB) (1999a) listed among the responsibilities of a supervisor of midwives that of ensuring that midwives have access to the statutory rules and guidance and local policies to inform their practice. This could be considered as 'nannying' (Stapleton et al. 1998) when the profession is self-regulated. Unfortunately, the experience of many supervisors (Duerden 1995, Stapleton et al. 1998) has shown that there is still an expectation by midwives that information and guidance will be provided unprompted rather than upon request. A common cry of midwives when asked why they have not seen new guidelines, or a recent publication, is the defence that they were never given the relevant document. A good example of this is ignorance of recent reports from the Confidential Enquiry into Stillbirths and Deaths in Infancy (CESDI), even though the summaries and recommendations were published with the

Box 11.1 Improving Behaviour and Communication

A midwife might have been caring for a woman who was particularly demanding, and felt it very difficult to maintain high standards of professionalism and communication with her. She was, perhaps, challenging in her disrespectful behaviour, and the instinctive response to her was out of character and unprofessional which, at the time, may have seemed appropriate. However, upon reflection the midwife might feel somewhat sullied by this experience. Taking the time to discuss this situation with a supervisor of midwives gives the opportunity to reflect on the reasons for such behaviour – a very human response – and to consider how it could be avoided in the future. The supervisor would, no doubt, empathise with the midwife, reminding of the inevitability of responding instinctively and helping determine some key messages to prompt and remind the midwife how to behave in future.

UKCC Register. (*The Register* was the quarterly newsletter of the UKCC, replaced by NMC news from April 2002.) This meant that all midwives received a personal copy through their door, but during audits of supervision and midwifery practice (Yorkshire LSA 2001) there was complete denial by many midwives of ever having seen such a copy.

Similarly, the requirement of a supervisor to provide guidance on maintenance of registration seems also to fly in the face of professional self-regulation. This should be clear to every individual midwife but, again, there are always stories of midwives who fail to re-register with the NMC and find themselves unable to rely on the vicarious liability of their Trust. When not currently registered, a midwife is in breach of contract and out of work and pay until re-registered. This is a really serious situation, yet the blame has been laid at the feet of the supervisor of midwives by the midwives concerned (Stapleton et al. 1998), despite the fact that the registration fees reminder goes to the midwife and not the supervisor.

THE MIDWIFE/SUPERVISOR RELATIONSHIP

This relationship is key to successful supervision. The underlying principle must, however, be mutual respect. No one-sided relationship can be successful. Midwives can be quick to criticise their supervisor of midwives for lack of contact but, as the saying goes, 'it takes two to tango'. Supervisors of midwives often find themselves undertaking many supervisory responsibilities – especially supervisory reviews – in their own time. The frustration of making the effort to go into a maternity unit on one's day off to meet with a supervisee to find that no one has turned up can well be imagined. The current workload of all midwives makes such meetings incredibly hard to achieve by all parties, who have their own professional commitments.

There will always be situations where there is a lack of mutual respect within the supervisory relationship. This must be the marker for changing the supervisor. Without respect, the relationship has no potential to bear fruit. Midwives should be able to choose their own supervisor of midwives. Usually, a list is provided to all midwives and they are asked to select approximately three supervisors of midwives by whom they would be happy to be supervised. This gives the supervisors themselves an opportunity to choose as well, rather than having an imposed caseload. With such choices, the supervisory relationship should be positive and fruitful.

THE BENEFITS OF EFFECTIVE SUPERVISION FOR MIDWIVES

In this age of critical incident reporting and medical litigation, midwives can easily feel disempowered and afraid to provide women with the care they have chosen in fear of reprisal or something going wrong. Supervisors can engender confidence in midwives through the advice and support they provide by drawing on their own experience and training to become a supervisor of midwives. This is illustrated in Box 11.2.

Supervisors can act as advocates for midwives in such situations, but may also act as advocates for women being denied choice because of midwives' underlying fear of reprisal or litigation. By successfully empowering midwives through support and advocacy, women in turn are empowered confidently to give birth in their chosen environment within safe parameters.

Midwives can be seriously traumatised following involvement in a critical incident. There may have been loss of life of a baby or a mother. It is difficult to think of a situation more traumatic than a maternal death.

Box 11.2   Supporting Difficult Situations

A common concern for midwives, especially those based in the community, is when a woman makes her choice for her labour and birth that is outwith or even contrary to local policy. Water birth requests that do not fit local criteria are a common example. In such a situation, a midwife may find herself in considerable difficulty and will need the support of a supervisor. The supervisor of midwives will also be tied to Trust policy and would be in breach of contract if deliberately practising against Trust policy. The supervisor's immediate role is to advise the midwife to explain the policy to the woman and to encourage her to adhere to that arrangement, but she will also point out that it is not appropriate to force the woman to leave the water under protest. She must, therefore, ensure that the midwife has the skills required to support a birth in water should the woman refuse to leave the birthing pool.

The supervisor will also be available to support the midwife during and after the birth so that there is an opportunity to debrief and to record why the birth was not according to Trust policy.

Following such an event, the supervisor of midwives can provide instant support, listening and empathy. The supervisor can direct the midwife to a trained counsellor for skilled help, recognising that training for supervisors does not include counselling training (NMC 2002). Just knowing that there is someone in the Trust to turn to is very beneficial. The supervisor is then able to make regular contact after the event to ensure that the midwife is benefiting from counselling and able to work again in the unit without increased anxiety. An example is shown in Box 11.3.

There are many situations when midwives do not feel comfortable about making decisions because of their lack of expertise and knowledge base. An example is where women suffer from mental health problems. Midwives are aware of the associated risk factors and the knowledge from the fifth Confidential Enquiry in Maternal Deaths (CEMD) (Lewis and Drife 2001) that suicide is the greatest cause of maternal deaths puts a huge responsibility on midwives to provide appropriate support for such women. (See also Lewis and Drife 2004.) Midwives need their own support through this process from peers and supervisors of midwives (Sullivan et al. 2003).

The 2001 CEMD report highlighted another increasing cause of maternal death, that of murder – which is the greatest cause of maternal death in the United States (McFarlane et al. 2002). Domestic violence, therefore, provoked many more recommendations in the CEMD report to be implemented by midwives and, thankfully, more training is available for midwives to address this social problem and to assist midwives in tackling the uncomfortable task of encouraging women to disclose domestic abuse, without being able to offer any solutions for them once such a disclosure has been made (Price 2003). Such anxiety can be shared with a supervisor or the supervisor can arrange for training in helping women to disclose and suggesting appropriate referral systems.

Concerns about domestic violence may be accompanied by child protection concerns. Community midwives, in particular, find themselves more and more involved in child protection procedures (Fraser 2003). Supervision is all

---

Box 11.3   Support Following Critical Incidents

A woman was taken to theatre for an emergency Caesarean section and had a cardiac arrest whilst being anaesthetised. Intubation was complicated and resuscitation was prolonged and difficult. The baby was safely delivered surgically, but the woman had to be transferred to the Intensive Care Unit (ICU) where she subsequently died. The supervisor of midwives was called into the unit whilst the woman was in theatre and problems were evident. She arrived in the unit as the woman was being transferred to the ICU. Her first action was to call in other midwives to the unit to take over all the responsibilities of the midwives involved in the incident. She then invited the midwives and healthcare assistants to meet with her to debrief following the incident. The obstetricians, operating department assistants and anaesthetists asked that they might join in the discussion. There followed a full account from everyone involved into their part in the activities surrounding this incident. This discussion provided a clear and comprehensive background for everyone who needed to write a statement following the incident. No blame was laid at the feet of anyone, but full support was given and thanks to everyone for playing their part so efficiently in trying to save the life of both mother and baby.

The supervisor then contacted the named supervisors for the midwives concerned to ask them to provide individual support to the midwives. They were then supported in statement writing. The next evening, when the staff returned to work, the supervisor was there again to see that everyone was alright and able to work another night. She and her colleague supervisors offered follow-up support to all of the midwives involved. The support offered to the midwives, medical and ancillary staff by the supervisor following that incident is still spoken of positively by staff at the Trust and it sets the standard for supervision there.

about public safety and the midwife's own responsibility to ensure the continuing safety of babies mean that, where there are child protection issues, the midwife and supervisor of midwives may find themselves working together on one case with the Area Child Protection Team. This collaborative approach reminds the midwife that she is not alone in dealing with such stressful and difficult circumstances. Unfortunately, it is not uncommon for midwives to feel personally threatened when working with families where abuse is obvious and the supervisor of midwives will ensure that adequate support and protection are provided for the midwife.

ENHANCING QUALITY OF CARE THROUGH SUPERVISION

Supervisors of midwives enhance decision making and quality of care in many ways, such as by ensuring that evidence-based practice is the norm and where practice should be challenged. (Evidence-based practice is discussed in Chapter 3.) Supervisors can assist midwives in understanding the concept of evidence and ensuring that midwives know where and how to find evidence and to evaluate it adequately, learning the difference between poor- and high-quality studies (Duerden 2003). Similarly, supervisors can support midwives to make positive contributions to the decision making process (e.g. by initiating a review of current policy within their Trust in light of newly published evidence). This takes courage in medically dominated climates, so it sometimes means the supervisor of midwives acting as an advocate for the midwife trying to introduce a change of policy within a multidisciplinary group, especially where the current practice is not evidence-based. It is, after all, the supervisor of midwives', responsibility to protect the public and ensure the highest standards of care and professional practice by midwives.

Further evidence that supervisors of midwives are able to enrich decision making and enhance quality of care is through their contribution to clinical governance and risk management. Here, supervisors can ensure safe midwifery practice and encourage the midwives on their caseload with life-long learning. An example of this is shown in Box 11.4.

Supervisors can help to create an environment that supports the midwife's role and empowers practice through evidence-based decision making (ENB 1999a). Supervision can provide a formal focus of support and reflection through supervisory reviews to provide the midwife with a confidential review of individual professional development needs, as well as a reflection on practice over the preceding year. In the modern, busy working environment, personal time is often overlooked, but taking time out for discussions with a named supervisor of midwives for a supervisory review can be immensely valuable. It is an opportunity for midwives to take stock of their careers, consider their future and to identify goals and opportunities, seeking appropriate advice and guidance from their supervisor. The supervisor can guide and direct, but the midwife does the choosing and reflection. Where a midwife has demonstrated high standards of care and commitment, the supervisor can take the opportunity to provide positive feedback and congratulation.

Statutory supervision of midwives has contributed to clinical governance since its inception. Supervisors of midwives were able to demonstrate to Chief Executives, after the publication of First Class Service (DoH 1998), that they had actually been practising clinical

---

Box 11.4 Support Following a Medication Error

Drug errors often go unreported (Birch and Culshaw 2003). The fear of recrimination in the current culture of blame makes this understandable, although not defensible. An understanding response from a supervisor of midwives will make reporting easier and encourage midwives to report and identify ways of eliminating error in the future by changing processes and procedures and identifying unsafe practices.

governance for many years. Supervision fulfils all aspects of the clinical governance framework. These are shown in Box 11.5.

DEFINING SUPPORT FOR MIDWIVES

Knowing that there is someone always looking out for one might seem a simplistic viewpoint, but for many midwives having a supervisor who is readily available to chat through a worry, bounce off an idea and listen after a particularly difficult case, can make an enormous difference to their working lives. Just being ready to say 'well done' or even a short greeting whilst passing in the hospital corridor helps to remove the isolation of autonomous practice. (Autonomy in midwifery practice is discussed in greater depth in Chapter 1.) The responsibility thrust on a midwife once qualified is described as overwhelming, and it can be just as difficult for a midwife returning to midwifery practice, especially after a break of many years. Some describe the experience as a steep learning curve (Oldfield 2003). The contrast to practice of possibly over a decade ago will be significant, with the post-natal ward now being closely related to a busy surgical ward. A supervisor of midwives is the assessor for every midwife returning to practice and this role is crucial, not just for assessing the midwife's competency, but also for providing

support whilst easing back into a much changed practice. Box 11.6 provides an example of where this may be required.

A recently qualified midwife (McIntosh 2003) wrote of her confusion between being a midwife and 'doing midwifery'. The ideology of the midwife's role of being to be with women is described as being in complete contrast to the task-oriented work of today's midwife in a busy, understaffed maternity unit. A supervisor of midwives is not in a position to change the environment but, by allowing a midwife to reflect on current practice, can understand the reasons for the current status and consider what could be done to change the service, and how midwives could influence that change. Supervisors can assist midwives in feeling less isolated and stressed by situations faced in daily practice.

Preceptorship should be available for all newly qualified midwives for at least three months on taking up new posts (UKCC 2001) and on moving to a new area, but in units where staffing pressures mean 'all hands to the pump' such close working with a preceptor is often not possible – hence the greater need for reflection with a supervisor of midwives. In many Trusts now there is a supervisor of midwives who takes responsibility for all the newly appointed midwives for their first six months in the Trust, until they have had time

---

Box 11.5   Clinical Governance Functions Enhanced by Supervision

- modernising and strengthening professional self-regulation
- ensuring that practice is evidence-based
- learning the lessons of poor performance
- identifying and building on good practice
- assessing and minimising the risk of untoward events
- investigating problems as they arise and ensuring lessons are learned
- supporting midwives in delivering quality care

Box 11.6   Support Around Perinatal Loss

Much is written about the need for psychological support for women following perinatal loss (Read et al. 2003). Midwives are expected to provide appropriate support for women following loss, but the experience may impact on midwives as individuals, as mothers themselves who have previously experienced similar loss. A newly qualified midwife in particular would find the first experience of dealing with this type of situation extremely stressful. Again, using supervision for appropriate reflection and support following such events is recommended.

to get to know the other supervisors and choose someone that they feel secure and comfortable with. This means that there is a supervisor for every midwife from the first day of practice. Most guidelines for supervisors recommend a meeting within the first week of appointment, if not available on the first day.

SUPPORT DURING CHANGE

During periods of major change, supervisors of midwives can be the bedrock for support during this challenging period. Reconfigurations of maternity services have led to many midwives feeling very insecure and reluctant to move from the area that they have practised in for many years. For many, moving to a different site will pose difficulties for the whole family as travel arrangements must change, and childcare may suffer in the process. Although supervisors of midwives are unable to influence the change, they can demonstrate sympathy and understanding and provide a listening ear. Regular, informal contact during the period of change: before, during and after; helps midwives come to terms with their difficulties and to feel supported.

Once a change has been introduced, the vulnerability for the midwife continues, especially if two maternity units have merged as part of the reconfiguration. It is quite remarkable how different the cultures can be in each maternity unit (Stapleton et al. 1998) and bringing those cultures together produces enormous conflict during the first months of forming and storming. Midwives believe that the practice in their own unit was the best and only way of doing things, and working collaboratively seems unattainable for the first few months.

During such times, midwives may find it difficult to conceal their animosity. This may be apparent to those in their care. Sometimes it takes time for the supervisors to appreciate just how bad a situation is, but community midwives are the best people to consult in this situation, as they receive the feedback from women after they have gone home. In these situations, supervisors should listen to community midwives and take appropriate action. They can introduce team-building activities and also identify the protagonists who can be given an opportunity to meet with their named supervisor of midwives to talk through their issues and discuss their own insecurities. The supervisor can reflect back to the midwife the perceptions that have been made by women and colleagues. This is often done with good effect, as we are all poor at seeing ourselves as others see us. If done tactfully, thoughtfully and sensitively, such a meeting can pay dividends and help to produce healthier working relations and a more positive and comfortable environment for both women and midwives. Further use of reflection is discussed in Chapter 10.

Much attention has recently been paid to the problem of midwives leaving the profession (Ball et al. 2002). When the number of midwives practising in the UK reached an all-time low, the Royal College of Midwives (RCM) commissioned research to find out why midwives were not staying in the profession. The report (Ball et al. 2002) makes salutary reading as midwives find their work in the midwifery profession very stressful. Supervisors of midwives can help to alleviate that stress as long as they are asked to take time to listen to the midwives and their worries. Supervisors of midwives too are practising midwives, with their own individual concerns, but that should not deter a midwife from approaching a supervisor. The supervisor, in turn, has a named supervisor to go to when the need to unburden and share a concern arises. An example of this relates to the demands of a very busy caseload, as shown in Box 11.7.

TRUST AND CONFIDENTIALITY

Without trust in any relationship there can be little hope of success. There is also a need to know that there will be complete confidentiality. Unfortunately, in a female-dominated environment, where chatter is a mainstay of social activity during precious breaks, carelessness often creeps into conversations. Personal information is also given and exchanged in a

---

Box 11.7   How Safe is a Tired Midwife?

Caseload-holding midwives are usually very keen to care for the women on their caseload when in labour. Unfortunately, it is impossible to schedule such events, so some midwives are willing to continue beyond their rostered hours in order to stay and support women who are anxious to be supported by midwives they know. In such situations midwives may feel such a sense of obligation that they stay even when overtired. The question must then be asked 'How safe is a tired midwife?' (Miller 2002). Decision-making is inevitably impaired when over-tired, so the woman being cared for could be considered at risk. If midwives feel they have overstayed at a birth, they might benefit from a reflective meeting with their supervisor to discuss the implications from that event and for future practice.

'multitude of encounters' (Lewis 2003: 34), and it is easy to lose sight of the professional requirement to protect confidential information as required by the Code of Professional Conduct (NMC 2004a). Similarly, within the supervisory relationship, it is easy to speak inappropriately outside that relationship. Surprisingly, midwives can be the worst protagonists when anxious to defend their actions and give their own version of accounts following incidents and the follow-up supervisory action. Despite this, the supervisor of midwives is duty-bound to maintain confidentiality within the supervisory relationship at all times. Any personal information disclosed during a supervisory interview should never be disclosed, but there will inevitably be situations where some information must be imparted to others. If a midwife is to undertake supported practice following the identification of some learning deficiency, then the arrangement can remain confidential between the midwife and the mentor and supervisor. Unfortunately, if the situation is more serious demanding supervised practice (LSA/ENB 2001), then it is not so easy to maintain

confidentiality, as the midwife must at all times work with a supervisor of midwives. The detail need not be revealed, but it will be obvious to most that the midwife's practice is being supervised.

The Code of Professional Conduct (NMC 2004a) reminds us of our duty to protect confidential information about women, but supervisors need to translate that code into information about midwives. Just as midwives should constantly consider the many ways, usually innocently, that confidentiality may be lost about the women they care for (Lewis 2003), supervisors should use the same level of confidentiality for the midwives on their case load. Training for supervisors of midwives (NMC 2002) emphasises the need for confidentiality within the supervisory relationship and underpins the mutual respect essential within the supervisor–midwife relationship.

INVESTIGATING CRITICAL INCIDENTS

Incidents can be reported in many ways and, in the majority of trusts, there will be a local reporting system, usually involving the completion of an incident report form. The risk manager for the department will examine these forms. Within maternity departments the risk manager may be a supervisor of midwives. When an incident involves a midwife, the named supervisor of midwives for that midwife will be available as the midwife's advocate to provide support in writing a statement, should the incident be sufficiently serious. The supervisor can also assist the midwife in assisting with reflection on the incident and determining any knowledge gaps. Where such gaps are identified, the supervisor of midwives can provide learning opportunities to improve knowledge and, if necessary, arrange opportunities for working in new environments to increase experience in the relevant area of midwifery care.

Learning contracts are an appropriate tool when more than one learning need is identified. The midwife, mentor and named supervisor all sign up to this contract to agree learning and mentorship requirements. The supervisor of midwives will arrange to meet regularly with the midwife to monitor progress and provide encouragement through the period of mentorship and learning. With this amount of support the midwife should emerge as a confident practitioner rather than feeling persecuted following an incident or error.

The approach described above is referred to as supportive practice (LSA/ENB 2001) and should, as described earlier, be a confidential arrangement between the midwife and the supervisor. In contrast, supervised practice is more formal, and a professional recommendation made by a supervisor of midwives. It usually follows an investigation of a significant clinical incident or a history of recurrent impaired midwifery practice. Supervised practice should only be considered when the level of concern is such that a midwife's practice could warrant referral to the NMC Professional Conduct Committee (LSA/ENB 2001). In reaching this decision, the supervisor of midwives should be clear that there is objective and impartial evidence that the Midwives Rules and Standards (NMC, 2004b) have been breached.

MONITORING STANDARDS

The standards for supervision are set both locally within Local Supervising Authorities, nationally through the LSA National Forum (LSA Midwifery Officers 2001) and through the NMC. The LSA Midwifery Officers monitor these standards through regular audit. The supervisors themselves monitor standards for practice within maternity units. Where procedures and protocols for practice are not followed, the supervisors can take action to determine why they have not been followed.

Protocols, policies and guidelines are in place to govern the way in which care should be provided (Beresford 1999), but these terms are often confused and may be used interchangeably. A *protocol* is a written system for managing care that should include a plan for audit of that care. Most protocols are binding

on employees as they usually relate to the management of urgent, possibly life-threatening, conditions (Beresford 1999). An example is a protocol for the care of women with antepartum haemorrhage, but only guidelines would be used for the care of women in labour without complication. If midwives work outside a protocol they could be considered to be in breach of their employment contract, whilst guidelines, or procedures, are usually less specific and may be described as suggestions for practice that are provided to implement agreed standards (Duerden 2003). Policies are general principles or directions, usually without the mandatory approach for addressing an issue, but might be considered mandatory in some Trusts. They are often set at national level, such as the indicators of success in Changing Childbirth (DoH 1993). To avoid confusion it is essential that supervisors of midwives ensure that midwives clearly understand the different definitions.

Supervisors of midwives audit records to ensure that record-keeping standards (NMC, 2004c) are achieved. Most audits are at random, with the intention of picking up omissions and errors, where they occur, and feeding back to midwives appropriately. This should be done positively as well as negatively, so where a good standard of record keeping is consistently achieved by midwives they are informed of their high standard, and praised for it. Similarly, where there are poor standards, supervisors will contact the midwives concerned to guide them into improving and explaining the deficiencies and their implications. Feedback should be constructive. If given positively and constructively it is helpful, if neutral it is usually negative but when destructive it is always negative and this approach should always be avoided.

LIAISON AND COMMUNICATION

As the CESDI reports tell year on year, poor communication leads to tragedy. Similarly, within supervision, communication is an essential element of success. The midwife and supervisor meeting together for the first time is the beginning of the supervisory relationship, working together is progress and staying together is success. Pablo Cassals (1876–1973) said that the capacity to care is the thing that gives life its deepest significance. The capacity to care should be one of the strongest characteristics of a supervisor of midwives. Active listening by the supervisor should take up three-quarters of the time spent with a supervisee. A midwife benefiting from good supervision will feel validated and supported both as a person and as a worker.

ROLE MODELLING

When midwives were asked what were the most important characteristics of a supervisor of midwives (Duerden 1995), many thought being a role model was particularly important. This means that the supervisor of midwives must have high standards of professional practice, be an enthusiastic, motivated practitioner, able to smile in adversity, and willing to offer support. A supervisor of midwives should be wise, reliable, empowering, in-touch, up-to-date, a natural born leader and, by all accounts, a paragon! No one is perfect, nor equipped with all of these qualities, and to be a good role model does not mean that a supervisor should demonstrate all of these characteristics. A supervisor as a role model will need, however, some leadership qualities to be able to support and challenge midwives in equal measure.

SUMMARY

Supervision has changed beyond recognition in more than 100 years of its existence. Many would say that the most fundamental changes have taken place in the past decade (Hawkins 2002). Supervision has been modernised and recognised for the support it gives to midwives, alongside its role of protecting the public. The NMC and the Midwifery Committee are keen to ensure that supervision has a very high profile throughout the UK with consistent standards in each of the four countries (NMC 2003). The intention is to maintain a robust system of supervision throughout the midwifery profession, supported by LSAs.

An effort has been made to offer a practical approach to maximising the benefits of statutory supervision of midwives. A very helpful booklet was prepared by the English National Board (ENB 1999b) and is still recommended today. *Supervision in action* explains supervision and its benefits in a very readable format and should be read by every practising midwife, especially when newly qualified.

KEY POINTS FOR BEST PRACTICE

- Midwives, especially when newly qualified, would be wise to consider using their named supervisor of midwives to assist them with decision making.

- Midwives will use their own professional judgement based on their current knowledge and experience, but the confidence to make decisions using that knowledge base needs to be developed. The supervisor of midwives can assist with that development.

- A supervisor of midwives can encourage midwives to develop professional judgement and make clinical decisions (NMC 2002).

References

Ball L, Curtis P, Kirkham M 2002 Why do midwives leave? RCM, London.

Beresford G 1999 Defining Quality Assurance. In: Bennett VR, Brown LK (eds), Myles Textbook for Midwives, 13th edition. Churchill Livingstone, Edinburgh.

Birch L, Culshaw A 2003 Drug error in maternity care: a multi-professional issue. British Journal of Midwifery 11(3): 173–175.

Department of Health 1993 Changing childbirth: report of the expert maternity group. HMSO, London.

Department of Health 1998b First Class Service. HMSO, London.

Department of Health 2001a Establishing the new Nursing and Midwifery Council. April 2001.

Dowie J, Elstein A 1988 Professional Judgement: a reader in clinical decision making. Cambridge University Press, Cambridge.

Duerden JM 1995 Audit of the Supervision of Midwives in the North West Regional Health Authority. Salford Royal Hospitals NHS Trust DMI.

Duerden JM 2000 Audit of supervision of midwives. In: Kirkham M (ed), Developments in the Supervision of Midwives. Books for Midwives Press, Manchester.

Duerden JM 2003 Supervision of Midwives and Clinical Governance. In: Fraser D, Cooper M (eds), Myles Textbook for Midwives, 14th edition. Churchill Livingstone, Edinburgh.

English National Board for Nursing, Midwifery and Health Visiting (1999a) Advice and Guidance to Local Supervising Authorities and Supervisors of Midwives. ENB, London.

English National Board for Nursing, Midwifery and Health Visiting (1999b) Supervision in Action – a practical guide for midwives. ENB, London.

Fraser J 2003 A baby in need of protection. The Practising Midwife 6(3): 19–20.

Hawkins J 2002 Supervision is worth celebrating. The Practising Midwife 5(2): 4–5.

House of Commons 1902/1997 Nurses, Midwives and Health Visitors Act. HMSO, London.

Lewis G, Drife J (eds) 2001 Why Mothers Die 1997–1999. The Confidential Enquiries into Maternal Deaths in the UK. HMSO, London.

Lewis G, Drife J 2004 Confidential Enquiry into Maternal and Child Health; Why Mothers Die 2000–2002. Sixth Report of the Confidential Enquiries into Maternal Deaths in the UK. RCOG Press, London.

Lewis P 2003 Confidentiality. The Practising Midwife May 6(5): 34.

LSA Midwifery Officers England 2001 Statutory supervision of midwives national standards for England. LSAMO, London.

LSA Midwifery Officers England and English National Board (LSA/ENB) 2001 Guidance on Supervised Practice Programmes.

McFarlane J, Campbell JC, Sharps P, et al. 2002 Abuse during pregnancy and femicide: urgent implications for women's health. Obstetrics and Gynecology 100(1): 27–36.

McIntosh I 2003 Am I a midwife or am I "doing midwifery"? Midwifery Matters Autumn 96: 8–9.

Miller S 2002 How safe is a tired midwife? New Zealand College of Midwives Journal 27: 5–8.

Nursing and Midwifery Council 2002 Preparation of Supervisors of Midwives. McMillan-Scott, Borough Green.

Nursing and Midwifery Council 2003 NMC News Winter 2003 NMC Online. www.nmc-uk.org.

Nursing and Midwifery Council 2004a Code of Professional Conduct: standards for conduct, performance and ethics. NMC, London.

Nursing and Midwifery Council 2004b Midwives Rules and Standards. NMC, London.

Nursing and Midwifery Council 2004c Guidelines for Records and Record Keeping. NMC, London.

Oldfield T 2003 Returning to midwifery. Journal of Family Health Care 13(3): 63–64.

Price S 2003 Tackling domestic violence. The Practising Midwife 6(3): 15–18.

Read S, Stewart C, Cartwright P, Meigh S 2003 Psychological support for perinatal trauma and loss. British Journal of Midwifery 11(8): 484–488.

Richmond H 2003 Women's experience of waterbirth. The Practising Midwife 6(3): 26–31.

Stapleton H, Duerden J, Kirkham M 1998 Evaluation of the impact of The Supervision of Midwives on Professional Practice and The Quality of Midwifery Care. ENB, London.

Sullivan A, Raynor M, Oates M 2003 Why mothers die: perinatal mental health. British Journal of Midwifery 11(5): 310–312.

United Kingdom Central Council For Nursing Midwifery and Health Visiting 2001 Supporting nurse, midwives and health visitors through lifelong learning. UKCC, London.

Yorkshire LSA 2001 Audit of supervision and midwifery practice – reports from audits at each Trust in Yorkshire. LSA Office, Yorkshire.

Further Reading

English National Board for Nursing, Midwifery and Health Visiting (1999) Supervision in Action – a practical guide for midwives. ENB, London.

This useful booklet helps midwives to get the most out of supervision. It is very user friendly and explains the supervision of midwives very succinctly from the perspective of the midwife rather than the supervisor of midwives.

Kirkham M (ed) 1996 Supervision of Midwives. Books for Midwives Press, Cheshire.

This book contains a comprehensive examination of the supervision of midwives beginning with a fascinating history of supervision and also giving some examples of good practice within supervision.

Kirkham M (ed) 2000 Developments in the Supervision of Midwives. Books for Midwives Press, Manchester.

Following on from the previous book, this edition explores how the supervision of midwives has developed in recent years, describing research and audit of supervision, changes in practice and education and training for supervisors of midwives.

Stapleton H, Duerden J, Kirkham M 1998 Evaluation of the impact of The Supervision of Midwives on Professional Practice and The Quality of Midwifery Care. ENB, London.

This is the report of a large study of differing models of supervision practised in five very varied geographical areas in England. It describes how midwives evaluated their personal supervision and gives some challenging descriptions from punitive to supportive supervision.

Chapter **12**

Skilled Decision Making: The 'Blood Supply' of Midwifery Practice

Amanda Sullivan

INTRODUCTION

Decision making is fundamental to midwifery practice. It defines the profession as a whole, guides best practice, and influences the actions of all concerned. Midwifery decisions can be made following long periods of conscious reflection, or subconsciously in emergency situations. If midwives were without highly developed decision-making skills, the lives of mothers and babies would be at risk and midwifery would not be a profession. Midwives would be lay helpers, relegated to the periphery of healthcare provision. In other words, decision-making acumen is the blood supply of the midwifery profession.

Many topics have been discussed in detail within previous chapters, so this final chapter will outline key learning points and common themes that have emerged. These will then be used to identify a vision of decision-making skills for modern midwifery. Finally, challenges to skilled decision making and the way forward will be discussed.

OVERVIEW OF DECISION MAKING

Decision making is a highly complex process. Decisions are the result of many interactions between cultural and societal norms and values; theoretical and tacit knowledge and individual motivations. It is therefore no wonder that attempts to describe decisions in purely rational terms are subject to criticism and are difficult to apply in practice. Unsurprisingly, reasoning is not always explicit and can appear inconsistent. Decisions are frequently shown to be wrong with the benefit of hindsight.

Despite these complexities, professionals must be able to unpick, reflect upon and justify their decisions. The chapters within this book have described a broad range of contributory factors. These are outlined in the summary chart shown in Figure 12.1.

In Figure 12.1, factors influencing decision making have been themed into the categories of relationships, expertise and external influences. The factors included do not comprise an exhaustive list, and themes may overlap and interact. However, it is important for practitioners to be cognisant of these factors and to recognise how they may influence clinical decisions.

There are some important learning points from previous chapters that can help midwives to work effectively (Box 12.1). These learning points can help to define current decision-making requirements, and they can also inform future skills development.

EMERGING THEMES

It is apparent that decision making is the foundation of midwifery practice, although the complexities and skills involved are immense. Even so, effective decision making is not enough. Midwives are also required to facilitate parents' decisions about their care. This presents something of a paradox. Midwives must be capable of autonomous and informed clinical decision making whilst, at the same time, empowering others to make decisions about their care. In other words, midwives have to be autonomous and empowering at the same time.

DECISION MAKING AND PROFESSIONALISM

This has implications for all healthcare professions. Professions are accepted because of their credible knowledge base. Knowledge qualifies professionals to advise, to be autonomous, and to 'know better' than their clients (Williams 1993). Some kinds of knowledge are regarded

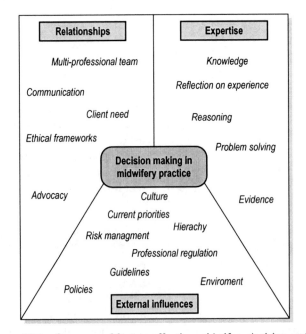

Figure 12.1   Summary of factors affecting midwifery decision making.

Box 12.1   Summary of Key Learning Points

- The level of midwives' decision-making autonomy is debatable. It appears to be exercised in a variety of ways. This can depend on local policy, culture and individual practitioners.
- Clinical knowledge can be theoretical and intuitive. The latter is difficult to describe, and its value is difficult to pinpoint.
- The ability to critically interpret and use evidence in practice is crucial to woman-centred care.
- Systematic clinical reasoning can help midwives successfully navigate unique and uncertain situations.
- When making decisions, all options should be considered. This can help to reduce the chance of errors occurring.
- Human information processing is subjective. It is biased and can appear inconsistent. This is because individuals interpret events according to their own values and beliefs.
- Individual interpretation of events means that opinions are often divided, even among experts.
- Student midwives have to acquire acceptable standards of professional judgement before they can enter the profession.
- Decision-making effectiveness can only be established retrospectively.
- Learning through experience requires reflection. The amount of learning that has taken place does not necessarily equate to length of service.
- Ethical frameworks form the basis of clinical decision making, often subconsciously.

as more professional than others. For instance, scientific knowledge is often considered to be more credible than practical, experiential knowledge. This is why midwifery, nursing and social work have traditionally been regarded as 'semi-professions.' They lacked a unique body of knowledge and much of their work is skills-based (Finlay 2000). Professionals must be more knowledgeable than the clients they serve. Indeed, many professionals derive great satisfaction when using professional knowledge to 'solve' difficult clinical problems and to steer clinical management.

Despite this, paternalistic consultation styles are no longer acceptable. The emphasis is on working in partnership with clients, recognising their personal expertise and perspective. There are a number of factors driving this change. These include rising educational standards, improvements in access to health information and declining deference to professionals as figures of authority (Coulter 2001). Consumerism is now a core theme of government health policy. Consumer pressure is used as a means of instigating quality improvements. Moreover, there is a commitment to extending client choice, information and the power of personal preference (Department of Health [DoH] 2003). Specific recommendations for the maternity services include access to midwives for first contact in pregnancy and promoting individualised birth plans. Client choice is no longer an optional extra.

It is evident that midwives must have a body of professional knowledge. It is also clear that professionals are increasingly called upon to surrender some of their decision-making autonomy and control to clients. This culture change is embraced by some, but there are also concerns about role erosion and diminished professional standing (Finlay 2000). So how can these seemingly opposing features of decision making be interpreted within the practice setting?

The bottom line is that clinical decisions must be shared. Professionals and clients have their own particular expertise. Furthermore, different professional groups have different perspectives. Professionals and clients each have a piece of the jigsaw that must be interconnected before the whole picture – and therefore the best decision – is apparent. Each must share information and negotiate with the other. Professionals have a view about relevant treatment options. Clients reveal information about lifestyle, personal values and preferences. Options can then be discussed within the context of client needs and values (Elwyn and Charles 2001). This means that current and future midwives must be equipped to face the challenges of redrawing professional boundaries, in order to adopt a more flexible approach to communication and decision making. Davies (1995) argues that caring professionals should engage with those in their care and should not be over-involved or detached. Professionals are also required to be reflective users of experience and expertise and not the master or keeper of knowledge.

SHARED DECISION MAKING

Shared decision making offers a way forward for healthcare professionals. It incorporates working in partnership with clients, promoting informed choice and negotiating a consensus decision. It can be viewed in three main stages:

1. Defining the clinical issue or problem.
2. Information giving about relevant options.
3. Deciding on the best course of action.

Defining the issue may involve clinical observations, history taking, making a diagnosis, or acknowledging expressed anxieties or queries. Professionals need the knowledge framework to know which questions should be asked, and they must also be able to identify salient points (O'Reilly 1993). Likewise, mothers should be facilitated to ask the questions that are relevant to their priorities and concerns (Entwistle and O'Donnell 2001). Midwifery decisions should be based on what is important for parents, as well as clinical issues identified by the midwife.

Once the problem or issue has been identified, future options become apparent and must be discussed. This can be regarded as the second stage of shared decision making. Midwives may share information in a variety of ways. Written information has been developed in relation to many aspects of maternity care. The Internet hosts a vast information resource, while pregnancy and childbirth are also commonly presented in the media. This plethora of information can be viewed as reducing the need for midwives to provide information themselves. In practice, it is more likely to generate new questions than to provide all the answers.

Ethical and legal frameworks underpinning midwifery practice recognise the rights of mothers to exercise informed choice. The communication of information about the risks and benefits of treatment options and consent policies are embedded in risk management standards (Clinical Negligence Scheme for Trusts [CNST] 2002). Unfortunately, the effectiveness of information-giving interventions is under-researched (Bekker et al. 1999, Briss et al. 2004). Although there is evidence that information increases knowledge, it is not clear whether this actually improves decision making (Briss et al. 2004).

The informing stage of shared decision making should help, and not hinder. It is sometimes believed that midwives should be non-directive when giving information, in order to reduce professional bias or imply coercion. This philosophy is deeply embedded in practice when discussing fetal anomaly testing in pregnancy (Andrews et al. 1994). Parents are given information about their options and then asked to make a choice on the basis of their personal circumstances or beliefs. This is appropriate, since procedures such as amniocentesis risk causing a miscarriage of a healthy baby. Conversely, midwives are asked to 'recommend' routine human immunodeficiency virus (HIV) testing because of public health concerns with vertical transmission rates (DoH 1999). However, it is appropriate to articulate judgements about the best option when these judgements can be supported by robust evidence (Elwyn and Charles 2001).

Adjusting the level of information to promote informed choice, without overwhelming parents, requires both skill and experience (Briss et al. 2004). If information is presented in a complex and incomprehensible manner, it is likely to increase anxiety and disengage parents from sharing in the decision-making process. Parents often want advice or recommendations and ask

"What would you do?" Karp (1983) referred to this as 'the terrible question' because one's personal decision is not a guide to the decision of other individuals. Recommendations are appropriate in some circumstances, so long as these are in line with evidence-based benefits and are neither coercive nor based on the midwife's personal values or beliefs.

The portrayal of health information and identification of options is also complicated by the fact that expert interpretations of the evidence may differ. Information can then appear to be conflicting. Disagreements may also arise concerning the amount of information and options that should be available. The promotion of informed choice is still not embedded within all routines and professions. One example is informed choice for antenatal anomaly scans, the delivery of which service many professionals are involved in.

Ultrasound poses a particular challenge for informed choice because it reveals such a broad range of suspected or actual problems. Parents do not always wish to know about problems such as Down's syndrome markers, even though they would wish to detect any structural or fatal abnormalities. This is compounded by the fact that many parents eagerly anticipate the scan procedure and regard it as a chance to visualise their eagerly awaited baby. Sadly, parents are sometimes faced with life or death decisions concerning their baby on the basis of ultrasound findings.

Fetal anomaly testing is controversial. Parents' views and personal choices should be respected, although these may not conform to routine procedures or the beliefs of professionals. Some differing priorities and perspectives in relation to ultrasound scan information are listed in Table 12.1. These perspectives can cross professional boundaries, but can sometimes result in disagreement and debate.

Differing approaches to information-giving, alongside the complexity of tailoring information to meet individual need, have contributed to much confusion concerning informed choice. However, there is a commitment to extending choice and effective strategies, and techniques for information giving will develop in time.

The third stage of shared decision making involves using the information to reach a decision about the way forward. This involves the midwife and parents working together to build a consensus agreement. There is joint responsibility for the decision that is made.

Table 12.1   Different Priorities and Perspectives Concerning Ultrasound Scans

Midwifery	Radiology
–Support for parents to make informed choices. –Fear of causing anxiety or spoiling the scan experience if too much pre-test information is given about potential abnormalities. –Limited time to discuss complex issues at booking.	–Perform examination and record findings. –Looking for suspected or definite abnormalities. –Report all findings. –Achieving good detection rates. –Main function is to perform the examination, not to discuss findings.

Parents	Obstetrics
–Looking forward to 'seeing' the baby. –May be anxious if previous experience of problems. –May wish to limit information received about certain problems (e.g. potential Down's syndrome). May only wish to know fatal conditions or instances when it is advantageous to plan surgery or requirements for birth.	–Scan provides useful information for pregnancy management. –Devise care management plans in relation to problems detected.

This is a compromise between paternalistic consultation styles and the non-directive approach to informed choice. The midwife can influence the decision without dominating the process. Parents also participate in decisions about their care, without feeling overwhelmed by the responsibility of the decision to be made (Quill and Brody 1996).

This means of decision making seems to offer a pragmatic 'third way' for clinical decision making, and should become an integral aspect of midwifery practice. It will require midwives to be systematic and articulate when making decisions, whilst having the confidence to influence and empower others to contribute. The need to articulate and document decision rationales is already recognised in practice. However, many chapters in this book allude to the fact that decision making does not always appear rational and that subconscious, intuitive processes also come into play. This phenomenon will now be explored in more detail.

INTUITION AND CLINICAL DECISION MAKING

Intuition is often referred to in midwifery practice. 'Gut feelings' may be used to justify a particular course of action. Furthermore, the spiritual connotations and profound nature of childbirth mean that 'women's intuition' has assumed some credibility. Some independent midwives in the United States regard this intuition to be authoritative knowledge. They believe their 'inner voice' should be listened to and trusted in preference to 'technomedical' knowledge (Davis-Floyd and Davis 1996).

Intuition is sometimes thought of as a mystical force that has no rational explanation (Brokensha 2002), although clinical intuition can also be seen as an interpretive process (Cioffi 1997). As such, intuitive judgements are said to be based on visual and verbal cues that are so rapidly observed that their contributions to the overall judgement are not remembered. In other words, it could be argued that intuitive decision making is subconscious pattern recognition that develops with experience. Accordingly, there is evidence that novices

adhere rigidly to taught plans or rules, whilst competent practitioners begin to see long-term goals and wider conceptual frameworks. Expert practitioners no longer rely explicitly on guidelines, rules or maxims (Greenhalgh 2002). This latter view of intuition as a feature of expert practice is now widely accepted within many healthcare professions, including medicine (Brokensha 2002).

Greenhalgh (2002) believes that it is time to reconcile intuition and evidence-based practice. Certainly, intuition is an integral part of midwifery practice. It is essential to combine the science and the art. Although it is difficult to define and evaluate the contribution of intuition to decision making, it is not impossible. One powerful tool is critical reflection. Intuitive thoughts can be recorded in relation to clinical incidents and outcomes. This will enable patterns to be detected and help develop tools for evaluation (Wickham 2001). Critical reflection also highlights areas of ambiguity, sharpens perceptual awareness, and exposes the role of emotions in decision making (Greenhalgh 2002).

CONCLUSION

This final chapter has taken an overview of midwifery decision making and has explored emerging themes in relation to current challenges for the profession. It is apparent from previous chapters that decision making is multifactoral and highly complex. Decision-making effectiveness is only apparent with hindsight. Decisions should encompass the wishes and perspectives of parents and other professions, alongside midwifery evidence and intuitive expertise. The skills required for this will be crucial to the development of midwifery. Pre- and post-registration programmes will need to equip midwives to deal with this challenge.

THE FUTURE

Current and future midwives need the confidence and skill to 'allow' parents to make decisions, even when they may not match professional recommendations (O'Reilly 1993). This may seem daunting, but practice norms and boundaries are dynamic. Today's ground-breaking decisions are likely to be tomorrow's 'bread and butter.' Midwifery practice is constantly evolving. For instance, in the past many midwives routinely hospitalised mothers with spontaneous rupture of membranes at term because of the 'dangers' of infection. These days, mothers without additional complications are 'allowed' to return home provided that they have clear liquor and their baby appears well. The value of electronic fetal monitoring has also been reassessed in the light of new evidence.

In the future, greater emphasis on decision-making acumen will be unavoidable, and the climate and culture of practice will need to respect and promote this. Education and skills development will be key facilitators. There is also a need for supportive professional boundaries that give midwives the confidence to take responsibility for decisions and then to share this responsibility with those in their care. In other words, there must be clear legal and clinical frameworks that support each stage of the shared decision-making framework, and they must be culturally embedded. If this is achieved, the impetus of 'Changing Childbirth'

(DoH 1993) can be restored. There will then be more choice for pregnant women, more and better information, more support for individual needs, and – all being well – better decisions.

KEY POINTS FOR BEST PRACTICE

- Clinical decision making is a defining feature of the midwifery profession.

- Midwives must be capable of autonomous and informed decision making, whilst empowering parents to make decisions about their care.

- Decisions must be defined, discussed and then made in collaboration with parents and other professionals.

- Promoting informed choice requires skill and experience, since parents have varying information requirements.

- Midwives can make recommendations so long as they are in line with evidence-based benefits and there is no coercion.

- Effective decision making involves the science (evidence) and the art (intuition) of midwifery.

References

Andrews L, Fullerton J, Holtzman N, et al. 1994 Assessing Genetic Risks. Implications for Health and Social Policy. National Academy Press, Washington, DC.

Bekker H, Thornton JG, Airey CM, et al. 1999 Informed decision making: an annotated bibliography and systematic review. Health Technology Assessment 3(1): 29–32.

Briss P, Rimer B, Reilley B, et al. 2004 Promoting informed choices about cancer screening in communities and healthcare systems. American Journal of Preventive Medicine 26(1): 67–80.

Brokensha G 2002 Clinical intuition: more than rational? Australian Prescriber 25(1): 4–5.

Cioffi J 1997 Heuristics, servants to intuition, in clinical decision making. Journal of Advanced Nursing 26: 203–208.

Clinical Negligence Scheme for Trusts 2002 Risk management standards for the maternity services. NHS Litigation Authority, UK.

Coulter A 2001 The future. In: Edwards A, Elwyn G (eds), Evidence-based Patient Choice. Inevitable or Impossible? Oxford University Press, Oxford, pp. 308–321.

Davies C 1995 Gender and the Professional Predicament in Nursing. Open University Press, Buckingham.

Davis-Floyd R, Davis E 1996 Intuition as authoritative knowledge in midwifery and home birth. Medical Anthropology Quarterly. Special edition 10(2): 237–269.

Department of Health 1993 Changing Childbirth: the report of the Expert Maternity Group. HMSO, London.

Department of Health 1999 Reducing mother to child transmission of HIV. Health Service Circular August 1999/183. HMSO, London.

Department of Health 2003 Building on the best. Choice, responsiveness and equity in the NHS. Stationery Office Ltd (TSO), UK.

Elwyn G, Charles C 2001 Shared decision making: the principles and the competences. In: Edwards A, Elwyn G (eds), Evidence-based Patient Choice. Inevitable or Impossible? Oxford University Press, Oxford, pp. 118–143.

Entwistle V, O'Donnell M 2001 Evidence-based healthcare: what roles for patients? In: Edwards A, Elwyn G (eds), Evidence-based Patient Choice. Inevitable or Impossible? Oxford University Press, Oxford, pp. 34–49.

Finlay L 2000 The challenge of professionalism. In: Brechin A, Brown H, Eby MA (eds), Critical Practice in Health and Social Care. Sage, London, pp. 73–95.

Greenhalgh T 2002 Uneasy bedfellows? – reconciling intuition and evidence based practice. British Journal of General Practice 52: 395–400.

Karp L 1983 The terrible question. American Journal of Medical Genetics 23: 359–362.

O'Reilly P 1993 Barriers to effective clinical decision making in nursing. Online. http://www.clininfo.health.nsw.au/hospolic/stvincents/1993/a04.html.

Quill TE, Brody H 1996 Professional recommendations and patient autonomy: finding a balance between professional power and patient choice. Annals of Internal Medicine 125: 763–769.

Wickham S 2001 Evidence informed midwifery 3: evaluating midwifery evidence. Online www.withwoman.co.uk/contents/evidence/dwknowledge.html.

Williams J 1993 What is a profession? Experience versus expertise. In: Walmsley J et al. (eds), Health,Welfare and Practice: Reflecting on Roles and Relationships. Sage, London, pp. 8–15.

Further Reading

Department of Health 2003 Building on the best. Choice, responsiveness and equity in the NHS. Stationery Office Ltd (TSO), UK.
This government document gives an overview of how choice and equity will be developed within the NHS. It presents the results of a large consultation on what choices should be available and how this should be delivered. It also covers the requirement for shared decision making in practice. There is a section on maternity services.

Eysenck M, Keane M 2000 Cognitive Psychology: A Student's Handbook, 4th edition. Psychology Press, UK.
This is a textbook for under-graduate psychology students. It contains understandable information about thought processes. In particular, there is a chapter on Judgement and Decision Making. An understanding of the psychological processes underpinning decision making can help midwives to analyse their own clinical decisions.

Glossary

A priori Before or independent of experience. *A priori* knowledge suggests we may know something without experiencing it. *A priori* statements are analytical and *true* based on logical rather than factual or empirical grounds; for example, the statement 'all triangles have three sides' is necessarily true.

Accountability Being answerable for any actions undertaken and/or omissions.

Assertive Self-confident in one's rights and opinions.

Authority The power or right to enforce obedience/delegated power.

Body of knowledge Knowledge deemed to be unique and exclusive to a particular profession that forms the fundamental nature of the profession itself, and could even provide the foundation for the ethos (morals, values, attitudes and beliefs) of the profession. This is why there is debate about whether nursing is a profession – as it takes most of its knowledge from medicine, sociology, psychology, etc. Midwifery has been included in this debate as taking knowledge from other professions – that is why the rationale that the unique relationship midwives have with the women they care for may support the argument that midwifery is a profession with a unique body of knowledge.

Bolam Standard This is where the action of negligence is linked to the standard of care expected from someone with skills and knowledge (the professional) against someone without these. (All England Law Reports 1957.)

Bolitho principle This differentiates between the actions of the professional and the expectation of excellence when the professional has been deemed an expert in that profession. This might be linked to their status in the form of their job title and the expectation of the level of care owed to the public as a result of this. (Bolitho v. City & Hackney Health Authority 1997.)

Clinical Negligence Scheme for Trusts (CNST) is administered by the National Health Services Litigation Committee (NHSLA); it is one of two schemes providing reimbursement to Trusts in relation to medical negligence claims. Its main framework relies on assessment of care to agreed standards and the mechanisms in place for the reporting and management of risk within the clinical setting.

Cognitive Intellectual knowledge – relating to the process of cognition or acquiring knowledge.

Compulsive Obsessive and habitual behaviour, contrary to one's conscious wishes.

Concept Mental impression or idea.

Conscience Moral sense of right and wrong.

Deduction Arriving at facts through reasoning from a general truth to a particular instance of that truth (e.g. all men are mortal; Charlie is a man; therefore Charlie is mortal). The deductive process is when inference is made from statements in which a necessarily true conclusion is arrived at by rules of logic (to state that Charlie is a man and then deny that he is mortal, is illogical given the premise in the first statement). Compare deduction with induction.

Deductive Drawing inferences from the facts, knowledge, experience and analysis in order to arrive at a valid judgment(s).

Deontology Duty-based theory, with followers observing one or more duties according to their school of thought.

Dilemmas Problems created by the conflict of principles, where all the choices offered seem to lack total satisfaction.

Duty of care A legal duty binding all people to consider the effects of their actions on others who could foreseeably be affected by them.

Empiricism In philosophical terms, it is a theory that all knowledge of matters of fact are based upon experience. Empirical enquiry would mean going out into the world and recording the data – in other words, the world is observable.

Epistemology Literally means the study of knowledge. Epistemological means about knowledge – a branch of philosophy concerned with the theory of knowledge. This chapter takes an epistemological perspective in that it is exploring how knowledge informs decision making in midwifery practice.

Ethics The science of morals, moral principles/standards and rules of conduct.

Evidence-based practice (EBP) Practice based on knowledge.

Gillick competence A three-stage standard laid down by Lord Fraser to judge the competence of a minor, whereby the minor must: (1) understand the circumstances that (s)he is in; (2) understand the possible options available; and (3) understand the consequences of each option.

Heuristic Mental rule-of-thumb.

Hypothetical Assumed or thought to exist; conjectural; speculative.

Hypothetico-deductive process This arises from the field of cognitive psychology, but taking a pragmatic view; it could be described as looking at the pros and cons of any given situation. The overall aim is to use the powers of deduction to assess the probability or likelihood of an event or outcome based on the available evidence. Where such evidence is from authoritative sources and research findings, this can then be seen to underpin the authority, or validity of the decision.

Impulsive Sudden tendency to act without any thought; hasty and impetuous behaviour.

Induction Reasoning from a part to a whole, from particular instances of something to a general statement about them, e.g. All observed Xs have the characteristic Y; therefore all Xs are Ys (or in other words – All swans that I have seen are white, therefore all swans are white). Induction can result in a conclusion that expresses something that goes beyond what is said in the premises; the conclusion does not follow with logical necessity from the premises.

Interprofessional Team Objective Structured Clinical Examination (ITOSCE) An approach to assessment of clinical competence in which the components of competence are assessed in a planned and structured way using simulations/examples from practice.

The various professionals work as a team to fulfil the requirements of the examination which should be assessed objectively.

Intuitive Understanding without a rationale.

Intuitive-Humanistic Subjective approach, naturalistic, holistic and subliminal judgement.

Meta-analysis This is a specific type of systematic review and a research process in its own right, which increases the precision of the overall result. All the available data accessed and reviewed are subjected to the scrutiny of statistical analysis or mathematical synthesis. The results from the various sources are combined with due recognition given to any particular strengths or weaknesses in the original paper.

Moral Concerns the rights and wrongs of everyday living.

National Institute for Clinical Excellence (NICE) A Special Health Authority set up to promote clinical and cost-effectiveness, through guidance and audit, and achieve consistent clinical standards across the NHS. First formed in 1999, this is part of the United Kingdom National Health Service (NHS) and its role is to provide a framework of best practice based on authoritative, robust and reliable guidance to patients and healthcare professionals. The guidance covers individual health technologies (fetal heart monitoring being one of these) as well as the management of specific conditions. Information about NICE can be found on its website: www.nice.org.

Paradigm Type of pattern; model or ideal theory.

Paternalistic Acting as if one knows what is best for another competent person.

Phenomenological Subjective, holistic, heuristic, non-measurable at time of decision.

Phenomenology Attributed initially to Husserl (1859–1938), a descriptive, introspective, in-depth analysis of all forms of consciousness and immediate experiences. Phenomenology studies and describes the intrinsic traits of phenomena as they reveal themselves to consciousness.

Positivism has a number of meanings. It may refer to the idea that the scientific method is the only source of correct knowledge about reality (there have been attempts to construct a unified system of all the sciences under one logico-mathematical/experiential methodology). In common-sense terms, this means trying to force the study of 'persons' or human nature into the framework of the natural sciences.

Praxis The individual has the capacity to act rationally, to think critically and to be self-reflective and therefore uses his or her knowledge of the world to control and manipulate objects but also to create knowledge. Praxis reflects the cognitive aspects of the person.

Prima facie At first sight.

Principlism Adherence to four main principles: autonomy, beneficence, non-maleficence, and justice.

Problem- or Enquiry-Based Learning (PBL or EBL) This is a recent development in midwifery education, and introduces the student to an identified problem or enquiry about which they are then asked to seek evidence for resolution or management. These models use clearly identifiable clinical situations in order to educate and stimulate enquiry that is based in the 'classroom' setting but relates to the clinical reality. This is in contrast to the conventional approach where there is a reliance on education based upon learning about care as a task-related entity and where these militate against the development of critical observation and enquiry.

Professional artistry The involvement of experiences of a more intuitive or reflective nature that are then applied to a different but similar set of circumstances with the aim of enriching the context within which a decision needs to be made. Information that will link to these sources of knowledge might arise from non-verbal behaviour, specific use of words and what has been described as 'ways of knowing'.

Rational Self-determining, self-controlled.

Rationalism The philosophical position that emphasizes reason as the primary source of knowledge, prior or superior to, and independent of sense perceptions.

Rationalist Clear thinking, which is not clouded by objective opinion and intuition.

Reasoning/intuitive approach This follows much the same pattern of assessing the situation with regard to probable outcome, but where what is observed, overtly and covertly (intuitively), is added into the equation along with existing knowledge about that individual or the circumstances surrounding an event. It then follows that the nature of the information used may be subject to interpretation about its validity and appropriateness.

Reflection An intellectual process by which the individual recaptures their experience, think about it, mulls it over, and evaluates it in order to lead to new understandings and appreciations.

Scope Sphere of action/the extent to which it is permissible to range one's practice.

Statutory Enacted, required, permitted by a written law of a legislative body.

Systematic Logical, sequential and objective; aimed at minimizing subjective elements. This is the key component of positivism.

Systematic review is a detailed and logical review process which collates all the available data, both published and unpublished, and then critically appraises them to enable conclusions for best practice to be drawn in the light of the available data and its quality.

Tacit Understood without being put into words.

Technical, rational perspectives This is the use or involvement of overt and quantifiable sources of knowledge as part of the information needs leading to judgements and decisions. This will include the use of chemical tests and values, of key physical measurements and characteristics which are not usually subject to any form of interpretation that would alter their original value. However, there may be aspects of how the evidence was obtained that might alter its meaning or reliability.

Utilitarianism Consequentialist theory, the goal being the greatest good for the greatest number of people.

Values What one considers to be good, desirable or important.

Index

Note - Page numbers in **bold** refer to figures and tables

Lightning Source UK Ltd.
Milton Keynes UK
UKOW010114040113

204370UK00003B/5/P

An Introduction to Health Psychology

Visit the *An Introduction to Health Psychology* Companion Website at **www.pearsoned.co.uk/morrison** to find valuable **student** learning material including:

- Multiple choice questions to test your learning
- Links to relevant sites on the web
- An online glossary to explain key terms
- Flashcards to test your understanding of key terms